A MANE
ATTRACTION

KAYE FLEWELLEN

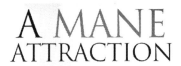

A MANE
ATTRACTION

Published by

KPI publishing
www.kpipublishing.com

Dallas, TX

Library of Congress Control Number: 2013915347

Cover design by Versus Company
Cover model: Ashley Kimbrae
Photographer: Blair Caldwell
Editor: Michelle Matthews-Calloway, Ph.D.

Dedication

This book is dedicated:
To my Mother, Mrs. Mary Flewellen for introducing me to her love affair with hair. She continues to be my mentor and motivation, and after nearly 60 years in the industry, she remains the most passionate person I have ever known in hair care.

To my brother, Edmond for teaching me how to dream and see all of the possibilities in the hair care industry.

To my only sister Sherry, for being such a Fashionista and raising the bar to show me the "Mastered Art of Hairstyling."

To all of my clients past and present for entrusting me with your "glory" and affording me the expertise I gained to write this book.

To all of my students, for being so eager to learn and inspiring me to avail my knowledge on a broader spectrum.

Special Thanks To:

Michelle Matthews-Calloway, Ph.D. and Ivy McGregor for pulling, and stretching me, holding me accountable and refusing to let me quit. It is true that iron sharpens iron.

Cora, for being my constant sounding board and my comic relief.

Marion (Cissy) Randel, the most reliable assistant one could ask for.

Rodney Barnett and Kim Avery for training the trainer. Your knowledge is invaluable.

Jill Waggoner, M.D., for all of your guidance through this project; and to my publicist Dena Craig, aka *The Fixer.*

A Mane Attraction: A Comprehensive Guide to a Healthy and Attractive Mane

Contents

Disclaimer: I am not a medical doctor or a pharmacist. The suggestions, recommendations or opinions expressed in this book do not constitute or represent medical consultation or treatment. Always consult your doctor or healthcare professional. The views expressed in this book are my opinion based on my exhaustive research on the subject and my own experience.

Forward

I Am Not My Hair . . . Or Am I?

Several years ago, soulful artist India Arie sang a song titled, *"I Am Not My Hair."* I am a big fan of India Arie. Her music is always so uplifting. So naturally, as a fan, when I first heard this song I was in love. It's not enough that I like her, but she had "the nerve" to sing about my favorite subject . . . HAIR. I listened to this song for several years, and with my head bobbing and fingers snapping I appreciated it every time. After all, it is masterfully arranged and it has meaning. A great song, indeed it was – until Easter Sunday, 2010.

In January 2010 I became ill. I was having problems with my blood. Severely anemic, I had to have several blood transfusions. I was prescribed a medication, and one of the possible side effects was hair loss. Being a diligent patient, I researched the medication and decided I'd follow my physician's treatment plan. After all, I am a stylist and I thought, "I know how to take care of my hair and if it sheds, I can handle a 'lil hair loss."

I began a process of using conditioners and a few home remedies I heard would be the silver bullet to ward off hair loss. Unfortunately, it didn't work. Soon I woke up to large patches of hair on my pillow. "Oh no, I never prepared myself for total hair loss," I thought. It was devastating!

If the disappointment of losing my hair was not enough, it was compounded by the fact that I am the "hair fixer - a gladiator." My job is to resolve hair issues. This shouldn't happen to me: I *fix* hair, not *lose* it. What did this say of my abilities? I wasn't a novice. At this point I already had more than 20 years of practice. I grew up in a hair salon. My Mom was a stylist and salon owner, and many of my childhood memories were either in the salon, on my way to the salon, just leaving the salon or at a hair show. My Mom still loves "all things hair," and serves as a point of reference and inspiration.

For icing on the disappointing cake of hair loss, we were heading into Easter Sunday and everyone had their hair looking good for Easter. After three days of sheer agony, on Easter Sunday I stood in my bathroom mirror and shaved my head. While many were off to celebrate the miracle of the resurrection, I was embracing what seemed in that moment to be the agony of the cross. I have had to do the "total chop" several times for clients and I always seemed to find the words to tell them it was gonna be alright. When the words were not directed at *me*, they always seemed to work. Somehow, all of those words eluded me in that moment.

Needless to say, that was the most difficult haircut I have ever had to do.

I've always been a student of my craft, but this was a pivotal moment in my life and career. My job is to facilitate all hair care needs, and obviously my hair was in need. Yet, I would not be defeated. I spent the next three months recovering physically and studying everything I could about hair, hair growth and hair loss. This information totally revolutionized my focus as a stylist. Now let me interject: I can still give you a "mean" haircut; but my focus shifted from just understanding the lines and angles of the latest cut to truly understanding hair.

I was off work for a few months recovering. During that time, I read everything I could about hair. I had more questions than a toddler who has just learned to ask "Why?" I had questions like, "Why do we have hair? What makes it grow? What makes it come out? How soon? How much?" and many more. With every answer I found, it seemed I had at least three more questions. I have always had questions about hair, and sought to find the answers, but when I lost *my* hair, my seeking became more intense. This is an interesting field with much to know. I will forever be a student of cosmetology and trichology, but my studies combined with over 20 years' experience and a lifetime of being in the hair industry have yielded many interesting facts.

Yes, I have learned much in my years of practice, but some of my wisdom comes from my Mom having over 50 years' experience as a licensed stylist, my brothers' 30 plus years in the industry coupled with my sister's 30 years doing hair. We share and bounce ideas off of one another. The result is a well-informed hair care resource. Much of the information I share with you in this book was gained on my quest for hair knowledge, from a lifetime spent in the business or from a first-hand understanding of the desperation to remedy hair loss.

Now, when I hear the song *"I Am Not My Hair"* I still enjoy it, and I certainly understand the message. I am so much *more* than my hair and skin - it is true that I am the soul that lives within. But maybe you can attest that if your hair is not right, it's the making of a BADDD day! Yes, you are much more than hair, nails, and skin. I know that those are just part of the packaging you are in; yet there is absolutely nothing wrong with presenting a gift in beautiful packaging.

For women, a full head of hair conveys beauty, femininity, and youthfulness. A beautiful healthy mane personifies sexiness. For men, a full head of hair represents strength, virility, youth and power. This is why a loss of hair often leads to frustration, depression, anger, low self-esteem, social withdrawal, and in extreme cases - suicide. It's not just about looks, although that's certainly a part of it; it's about a loss of control, our perception of our image and what that image conveys to others. Hair loss even reminds us of the inevitable - our mortality.

Extreme hair loss, like in the case of chemotherapy, often can lead to paralyzing sorrow and distress. In fact, some women have said that the mental anguish of losing their hair is as devastating as the actual therapy. In a study conducted in 2006 entitled "Post-Menopausal Women With Breast Cancer," by researchers Browall, Johansson, and Danielson, some women reported that the loss of hair as a result of the chemotherapy was worse than losing a breast.[1] Again I say, I know that we are more than our hair, but the emotional and psychological attachment to our hair is *real*. The Bible would go on to say that a women's hair is her glory; who am I to disagree? The question that follows is, "How do I maintain my glory?" How do I prevent hair loss?

Maybe your case is not as severe as a patient undergoing chemotherapy, yet for you, your struggle is just as real. Whether you want to restore the vitality and luminosity to your hair or simply maintain your crown and glory, you need a road map. In *A Mane Attraction* I will explain healthy hair, help you understand what it takes to get it, explore some health issues that retard growth, debunk some of the myths about hair care and offer some styling and maintenance tips that will help keep your mane attractive. Throughout the book you'll also see that I've assembled some of the best in the business from cosmetology to medicine to weigh in and provide expert input. From cradle cap to menopause, from the foods you eat to nourish your hair, to the products you use on your hair; this book explores common concerns and offers solutions to problems that impede hair health at any age.

What does your hair say of you? Does your hair tell a story of health, wellness and success – or does it sing a song of despair? I seek to tackle the psychology of hair. I hope to use my lifelong journey of hair exploration to empower you to have better hair days. I have a great appreciation for both knowledge and art. When they collide it is majestic! *A Mane Attraction* is a pre-eminent encounter of knowledge and art.

God made each of us beautiful, but as an artist, I have the opportunity to help you own your beauty!

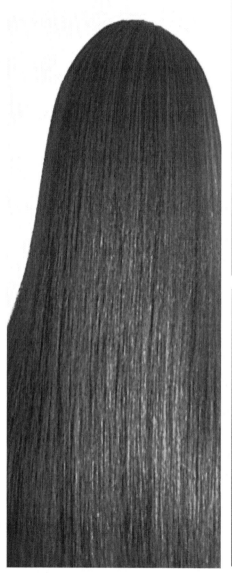

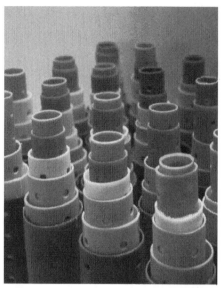

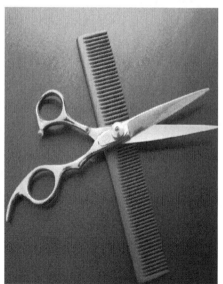

Chapter I
Getting to the Root of the Matter

I realize that if you are reading this book, you are likely anxious to discover answers to your hair questions. You may be tempted to jump right to the part about conditioners, vitamins or some of the other topics that you may find interesting. When new students come in my class on the first day of each semester, they always want to know how long before we start coloring or cutting hair. It is natural to want to start at the top.

Styling hair is fun, but before we delve too deeply into styling matters, let's take a moment to talk about hair and its structure. We need to get to the root of the matter. With anything, it is important to have a solid foundation. Let's start with a brief trichology lesson to help you understand more about your hair and how it grows.

Trichology is the scientific study of hair and its diseases. **Hair** is an elastic filament made up of keratin protein. The body is covered with hair. Hair was purposed for warmth and protection for the body. Some scientists believe that the hair on our head is nature's way of protecting and insulating the skull and brain. However, hair does help to regulate the body's temperature. We have two types of hair: *Vellus hair*, which is the extremely fine hair that has no pigment and covers the entire body except the palm of the hands and the soles of the feet. *Vellus* hair helps to evaporate perspiration and cool the skin. *Terminal hair,* which is the second type, is the longer, coarser, pigmented hair found on the head, eyebrows and eyelashes, arms and legs. For the purpose of this book, we will talk about *terminal* hair.

A strand of hair is divided into two parts: The **hair root**; the part of the hair that lies below the scalp or the surface of the skin. Only the root which is located in the *dermis*, is alive. **Hair follicles** are tubular cavities in the scalp containing the root of the hair; which is where hair is nourished and growth

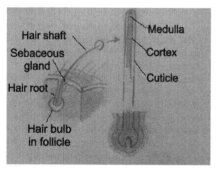
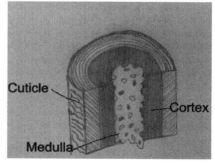

occurs. Each follicle measures about 3 to 4 millimeters in length. The **hair shaft** is the part that you see above the scalp (**See**

photo). It endures all of the harsh treatment both from the environment and self-induced factors. There are three layers in a strand of hair. The *cuticle layer* is the outer layer of hair that protects the inner layers from temperature changes, absorption of moisture (porosity), rubbing and pulling. It is the outside armor or protective barrier on hair.

The cuticle layer is comprised of many tiny, overlapping scale-like cells resembling the shingles on a roof or a

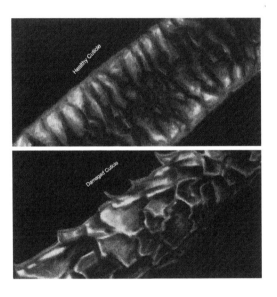

pinecone (**See photo**). In a healthy cuticle, the scales are tightly compacted and protect the inner layers from moisture and damage. When the cuticle is raised, hair is more susceptible to damage and dryness. The cuticle layer is also responsible for shiny, smooth and silky-feeling hair. In fact when hair is damaged, most of the damage is in the cuticle layer.

The *cortex* is the middle layer of hair. It is responsible for 90% of the hairs weight, keratin protein (strength), melanin (color), elasticity and curl. Like a tree, most of the moisture lies in the middle layer (cortex), behind a strong outer layer of protection. The *medulla* is the innermost layer of hair. The medulla is not engaged in the styling services. Some believe that all hair does not have a medulla. However, hair starts with a medulla, although it is very minute in some hair types, it is always present.

*Trichologist **Rodney Barnett** offers the following acronym to help you understand the seven properties of a healthy hair shaft:*

OPEN MAP: **O**il, **P**rotein, **E**lasticity, **N**atural Sheen, **M**oisture Balance, **A**cid Balance, and **P**orosity.

Oil. Below the hair shaft and under the epidermis are tiny glands called the *sebaceous glands.* These glands produce *sebum*, which acts as a natural lubricant or oil for hair and skin. It keeps the hair shiny and smooth and the scalp healthy. Chemicals, heated tools and environmental stressors can strip the hair of its natural oils. Replacing this oil is vitally important to keep hair pliable and vibrant.

Protein compromises approximately 90% of the hair shaft. Some researchers believe that as much as 97% of the hair shaft is protein. Protein is a hard substance that gives hair its structure, but it must be balanced with moisture. Chemically treated hair that is weak and fragile has compromised the protein in the hair. A protein treatment is recommended to restore the hair.

Elasticity is the ability of the hair to stretch and return back to its original place without breaking. It is important to determine the elasticity of the hair to judge the health of the hair and to determine if it is strong enough to accept chemicals. Chemically processing the hair can reduce the elasticity of the hair, sometimes as much as 25%. Hair with no elasticity is really fragile and prone to breakage.

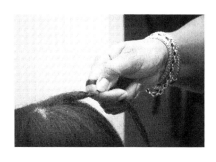

To test for elasticity, wrap a few strands of hair around the forefinger and gently stretch the hair about 10% (give the hair a gentle pull). Hair should return to its original position. If the hair sheds or pulls out, the elasticity is poor. To build the hair, protein conditioners are recommended. If the hair remains in the head, but fails to return to its original position, the elasticity is compromised to a degree and conditioning treatments are recommended. If the hair goes back to its original position, the elasticity is strong **(See photo)**.

Natural Sheen is the ability of the hair to reflect light. This works particularly well when the cuticle is smooth and even. When the cuticle is roughened by excessive rubbing or brushing, harsh chemicals and heat, the hair will not reflect its natural luster. Straight hair tends to reflect this sheen better. Diet and maintenance are crucial for maintaining this sheen.

Moisture Balance is a goal for all hair. Some hair types are prone to dryness and there is a constant struggle to add moisture to keep the hair shiny and free from breakage. Hair that lacks moisture is prone to brittleness, dullness and lifelessness. Those with excessively oily hair also face struggles, because hair that is excessively oily is stringy, limp, and difficult to style. Excessively oily hair often looks greasy and unclean.

Acid Balance refers to pH. Potential Hydrogen, or pH, is the measurement of how acidic or alkali a substance is. The scale ranges from 0 to 14 with 0 being a very strong acid and 14 being a very strong alkali. Both strong acids and alkalis should be avoided as they are hazardous for the hair and skin. Anything between 0 and 6.9 is acidic; 7 is neutral, and anything between 7.1 and 14 is alkaline. Human hair has a pH balance of between 4.5 and 5.5; water has a pH of approximately seven. The natural acidity inherent in hair prevents fungi and bacteria in the hair and scalp, and keeps the cuticle closed and healthy.

All products that are water soluble have a pH (including water) and can alter the natural pH of hair. A substance that is alkaline, like perms, relaxers, hair color and even shampoos will cause the hair cuticle to open. On the other hand, a substance that is acidic, like most conditioners will cause the cuticle to contract. Keeping the pH of hair balanced and as close to its natural pH is important to maintaining optimal hair health.

Porosity is the ability of the hair to absorb moisture and is directly related to the health of the hair. Porosity is identified as *low*, *normal*, and *high*. Normal porosity is ideal. Normal porosity has a cuticle that is slightly raised so the hair can absorb moisture, but it can lose moisture if it is not replenished often with conditioners. When the cuticle is tightly compacted, hair is considered to have low porosity and does not absorb moisture. The more porous the hair is; the more it swells and absorbs liquids. Hair with high porosity is often referred to as an *open cuticle*. The result is dull, dry, brittle hair that breaks easily.

How can you determine whether or not your hair is highly porous? There are many ways to test porosity. The most common is to conduct a "floating hair test." Take a couple of strands of your hair and drop them into a bowl of water. Let them sit in the bowl for about two to four minutes. Observe your hair. If you hair is floating in the water, you have low porosity. If your hair is sinking, you have high porosity.

This is not always accurate, because all hair has some level of porosity and eventually it will start to absorb water and sink. As well, if the hair has any product on it, it seals the cuticle and makes the hair slow to absorb the water.

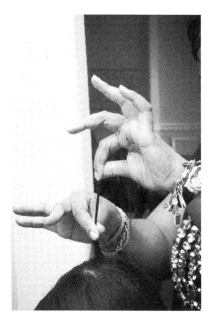 A better way to check for porosity is to take the several strands of dry hair. Hold the strands securely with one hand while using the thumb and forefinger of the other hand to slide down to the scalp **(See Photo)**. If the hair is smooth and without frizzes the hair has low porosity and is thus extremely resistant to moisture. Normal porosity will be indicated by minimal frizz in the hair. If the hair feels rough, is badly frizzed or even breaks, the hair has high porosity and has likely been over-processed. A balance of moisturizing conditioners and protein conditioners to fill in the gaps of the cuticle is recommended. Extreme caution is recommended when applying chemicals to hair with high porosity.

Note: Hair that swells and/or frizzes at the smallest amount if humidity is highly porous.

23

Number of hairs

Approximately 100,000-200,000 strands of hair can be found on the average head, with the number varying, sometimes dramatically, from person to person. A correlation exists between hair color and the number of strands on a head. Lighter hair is usually finer but more plentiful. Natural blondes average 140,000 strands. Darker hair tends to have thicker stands but less density. Brunettes and people with black hair average 108,000 strands and red heads average 90,000 strands.

On average, Hair grows about 1/2 inch per month for two to six years, and then rests for about three months. Male hair tends to be denser and grows at a slightly faster rate than females. On the other hand, eyebrows and eyelashes grow for 10 weeks and then rest for nine months. At the end of the rest cycle the hairs fall out.

At any given time about 90 percent of the hairs on a head are growing, while 10 percent of the hairs are testing. Shedding 50-100 strands of hair a day is normal. However, stress as well as health and emotional conditions can make your hair fall out at a more rapid pace. Excessive hair loss is an indicator of a bigger problem. (We will explore those problems later in this book). Hair grows quickest in young women adults between 16 and 24. It also grows faster in the spring and summer than in the winter and fall.

*Trichologist **Rodney Barnett** provides the following information about the growth cycle of hair:*

The Hair Growth Cycle
~Rodney Barnett

The hair growth cycle includes three phases, known as the anagen, catagen and telogen phase. The anagen phase is the longest, lasting between two and eight years. During the anagen phase the hair grows actively from matrix cells in the bulb, where the derma papilla is nourished by blood vessels.

The next phase of the growth cycle is the catagen phase. This is a short, two-to-four week transitional period in which the hair stops growing, and the lower portion of the hair follicle retracts up to the level of the arrector pili muscle. The dermal papilla is pulled until it breaks away and regresses, detaching the upper portion of the follicle from the blood supply. At this point, the hair stops growing.

The last phase of the growth cycle, the telogen or resting phase, lasts two-to-four months while the dermal papilla is in a resting state. Following the telogen phase, the hair follicle reattaches to the dermal papilla and the follicle re-enters the anogen phase. As the new hair begins to grow, the old hair is pushed out of the hair follicle. ♥~RB

This has been a brief lesson in hair and how it works. Refer to this chapter as often as you need. We will move on to other topics, but the information in this chapter should prove to be invaluable because it will help you to make more informed decisions about your hair, and enable you not to be easily persuaded by clever marketing seeking to sell you products not designed for your hair type. The foundational information presented in this chapter will serve as a basis for understanding the following chapters.

Note: Throughout the book, interesting hair facts will be provided in "Kaye's Klips." Pay special attention to these factoids because they'll help you learn even more!

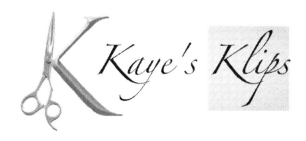

When dead skin cells and debris clog the hair follicles and make it difficult for hair to grow out of the follicle; the result is often ingrown hairs. Ingrown hairs are hairs that have curled around and grown back into your skin instead of rising up from it.

Although anyone can get ingrown hairs, they are more common in people with curly hair. Ingrown hairs are not a serious condition, but they can be unsightly and uncomfortable. Razor bumps, or pseudo folliculitis, is a cluster of bumps on the skin caused by sharp hairs trapped under the skin. This is a common manifestation of ingrown hairs.

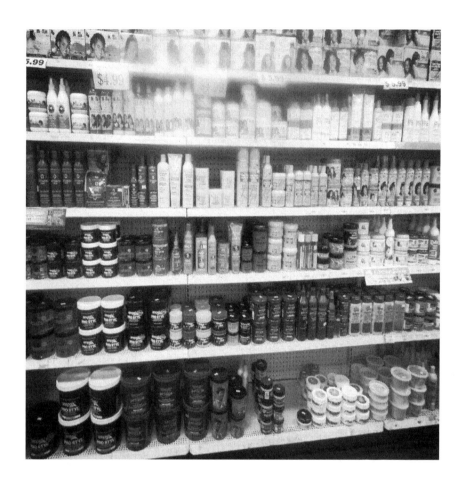

Chapter II
Healthy Hair - The Mane Thing

I recently had an opportunity to visit an ancient Egyptian exhibit featuring many artifacts from the King Tut dynasty. Evident from the display was the fact that the artistry of hair dates back to as early as ancient Egypt. Some reports suggest hair artistry goes back as far as the Ice Ages.

Since its beginnings, hair and its care has gone through quite an evolution; from the use of hair color by the Romans to indicate social class, to the towering headdresses and ornate hairstyles of the Middle Ages. With the invention of motion pictures in the early 20th century came a dramatic shift in our personal grooming practices.

Today a great deal of attention is given to our hair and its health. In 2003, analysts at Goldman Sachs estimated that $38 billion was spent on hair care products, with a growth rate of up to 7 percent. The global beauty industry has consistently experienced compound growths in profit. Some analysts have estimated the hair care industry has reached upwards of $60 billion annually. [2]

Much time, money and attention has been given to hair throughout the ages. Is it because hair is an important component of body image? Yes! Hair is one of few physical characteristics we can change and manipulate to our personal expression of beauty.

In her book, *You've Only Got Three Seconds*; Camille Livingston describes what happens in the first three seconds of meeting someone. [3] According to Camille, we make an assessment of what we believe to be a person's intellect, socio-economic background based solely on a person's image, and we look for evidence that we have something in common. Interestingly enough, our hair is a key component of this evaluation process. How you wear your hair says a lot to others about you. For this reason, your hairstyle will either attract or repel potential business partners and social acquaintances.

We are all unique, and each of us has our personal definition of style, fashion and beauty. Even so, the one thing that remains constant is everyone wants healthy hair. Healthy hair speaks to your physical well-being and your personal grooming habits make others feel comfortable with you.

The question becomes: "What is healthy hair and how does one obtain it?" I'm sure you don't need a dictionary to identify healthy hair when you see it. **Healthy hair** is strong - resistant to breakage, slightly porous, and elastic. Healthy hair is also soft, with buoyance and shine. By contrast, **unhealthy/damaged hair** has a rough texture; is dull, dry, and brittle to the touch. It also breaks easily, and is spongy or very porous.

A **healthy** strand of human hair is stronger than a strand of copper the same width. Even with its strength, hair should closely resemble the luster and luxury of silk. The molecular structure of silk is the closest natural fiber to human hair. Human hair has 19 amino acids and silk has 18 of those same amino acids. Therefore, silk and hair possess similar qualities. They are each strong and durable, yet soft and flexible.

Both silk and hair has good tensile strength, which allows it to be stretched 15 to 20% of its length without breaking. Wet hair should be able to stretch about 50% without breaking. It returns to its size without losing its shape. Silk is sensitive to heat and like hair, it begins to decompose at 350 F. Silk is also mostly comprised of protein which contributes to its porosity and allows it to be dyed, printed and stained much in the same manner as coloring hair. Lastly, both silk and hair are sensitive to extreme sunlight, excessive perspiration and harsh detergents. It is safe to say, you should treat your hair with the same or better delicacy as you would treat your silks.

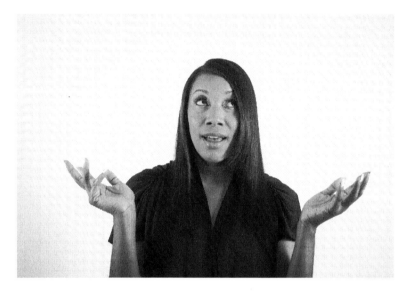

The question yet remains, **"How does one achieve healthy hair?"** The average woman spends approximately $1200 annually on hair grooming and this doesn't include the extra money spent buying maintenance products. Men invest only a fraction of that, spending an average of $300 annually on their hair, which does include any additional grooming products. Despite this level of spending, 1/3 of American women suffer from breakage, shedding, balding or some form of hair loss or alopecia and 70% of men suffer from Male Pattern Baldness.[4]

We are making the investment in our hair, but clearly the solution is not based solely in our investment. The answer is not as cut and dried as it may seem. **The bottom line is that four contributing factors determine healthy hair:** Genetics, Diet, Products and Routine Maintenance. Let's take a look at the role each of these factors plays in overall hair health.

Genetics

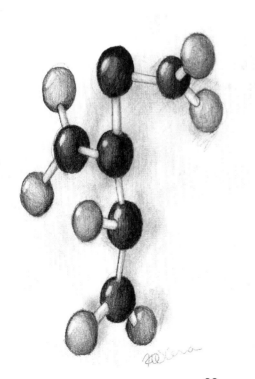

Human hair is composed of 19 amino acids and 11 of those are inherent. The body is able to produce them without any real help from you. These inherent genes will determine our hair color, texture, density and growth cycle.

Hair color is determined genetically by pigmentation of the hair from melanin. There are two types of melanin; first, *eumelanin* which determines the darkness. *Eumelanin* gives hair its amount of black or brown.

The second type of melanin is *pheomelanin*, which gives hair it lighter hues of yellow and orange. The amount of *eumelanin* or *pheomelanin* an individual possesses is totally determined by one's gene pool. People with more *pheomelanin* have lighter hair, and people with more *eumelanin* have darker hair. Although your hair color is determined genetically, the color can be slightly altered by physical and environmental factors. Although extreme stress and sickness can speed up the loss of melanin, the lack of melanin (premature grey) is also a genetic trait.

Texture measures the size of each hair strand. Because texture can vary from strand to strand, it also describes the overall *feel* of the hair. Texture is measured as *fine, medium* and *coarse*. *Fine* hair has the smallest diameter and as a result it is weaker or more fragile. *Medium* texture has a slightly larger diameter and is the most common. *Coarse* has the largest diameter and is the strongest.

Understanding texture is important, because it helps you to determine the amount of heat and chemicals the hair can take.

Density refers to thickness or the number of hairs on a head. Density is described as the number of hairs per square inch of the head. I'm often asked if there is something you can take or do to make your hair thicker. Unfortunately, density is determined by genetics.

To measure density, you could part your hair using a rat-tail comb. Gently pull hair back into a ponytail. If the part remains the width of the tail of the comb, you have medium density. If the part appears to be closing or very little scalp is showing it means your hair has high density. If the part seems really wide or if you see a lot of scalp, it means your hair has low density.

Growth Cycle is another factor determined by genetics. As mentioned earlier, a strand of hair is on your head from 2-6 years. That's a large gap, but the lifespan of a strand of hair is determined by genetics. Diet and maintenance can extend the lifespan of a strand of hair to a certain extent. Additionally, hair grows on average 1/2 inch a month. Obviously some people's hair grows a bit more and others a little less. The rate at which *your* hair grows is inherited. Hair growth can be slightly enhanced by a healthy diet.

Hair loss can be passed down from generation to generation, but not only from the mother's side of the family as the old wives' tale dictates. Genetically, *both* parents are responsible for hair growth, or the lack thereof. Hereditary hair loss can come from either side of your family. While hair loss can be due to your genes, many other factors could set it off, including stress, an unhealthy diet, sickness, poor use of products or poor maintenance. Let's take a look at some of these factors before you start to blame the family!

Diet

At times I found it hard to understand the statement, "You are what you eat." Yet, when it comes to your hair this saying is true. Contrary to popular belief there is **no** magic pill, potion, salve or formula for hair growth. Hair grows from within. Hair is nourished through the blood stream. The foods we eat are digested and used to sustain life of course; but these foods are also used to nourish the hair, skin and nails. Just like every other part of the body, the cells that support healthy hair depends on a healthy diet.

Your body has a priority system. If it only has a limited number of nutrients, your body sends those nutrients to the cells essential for life. A healthy hair diet would be one that includes Protein, Iron, Omega-3 Fatty Acids, Biotin, Zinc, Vitamins A, B, C, D and E and water.

Certified Pharmacist Charlene Shelby shared the following information on vitamins and corresponding food sources to describe how they react in the body to promote hair growth:

Vitamins and Your Hair
~Charlene Shelby, Certified Pharmacist

Protein

Proper hair nutrition begins with getting enough protein. Hair is comprised mostly of protein. Protein provides structure to the hair just as bones provide structure to the body. A diet that lacks sufficient amounts of proteins can lead to weak brittle hair, or fragile hair that lacks structure. A lack of protein also makes it difficult for new hair to grow. At any given time, about 90% of your hair is in the anagen, or growing phase. If you don't get enough protein in your diet, a disproportionate number of hairs may go into the telogen, or resting phase. *Food Source: Poultry, Fish, Beef, Pork, Tofu and Eggs*

Iron

Iron helps to carry oxygen to the hair follicles, which is vital to sustain hair. Like everything in nature the hair follicles need a sufficient flow of oxygen. We know that lack of iron leads to hair loss or thinning. Research determined that while all hair loss is not because of a lack of iron, hair loss is often exacerbated by low iron levels. Even mild cases of anemia can cause hair loss. Including iron in your diet will help keep your tresses full.

Food Source: Liver, Spinach, Lean Red Meat, Egg Yolks, Beans, Soybeans, Lentils and Artichokes

Omega-3 Fatty Acids

Omega-3 helps in the production of natural oils which combats dry and brittle hair, dry, flaky scalp and reduced circulation to the scalp, and hair loss. Omega-3s provide a much-needed boost by adding luster, sheen and elasticity to your hair and nourishing hair follicles. Although they critically improve the appearance of hair, the body can't produce the fatty acids necessary for hair health. We must consume these fatty acids in our diet.

Food Source: Seafood, Walnuts, Flaxseed, Pumpkin Seeds and Canola Oil

Biotin

Biotin is credited for buoyancy in hair and often called the hair growth vitamin. This vitamin produces keratin protein, the building block of hair. Biotin is a naturally occurring B-vitamin. Sometimes it's called vitamin H. Biotin is produced naturally in the intestines. Although deficiencies are rare, a lack of Biotin can lead to brittle hair.

Food Source: Nuts, Leafy Green Vegetables and Liver

Zinc

Zinc is essential for scalp health. It helps to prevent dry, flaky and itchy scalp. A lack of Zinc can also cause hair loss.

Food Source: Oysters, Lamb, Beef and Nuts

Vitamins

Vitamin A

The antioxidant beta-carotene is not a nutrient of itself, but your body turns it into Vitamin A. Every cell in the body needs this vitamin, including the cells necessary for hair growth. Vitamin A helps to produce the healthy sebum in the scalp. This moisture or sebum protects both your hair and scalp. The absence of Vitamin A can leave your scalp dry, itchy and even flaky.

Food Source: Orange foods - Sweet potatoes, Peaches, Carrots, Cantaloupe, Pumpkin, Mangos, Oranges and Apricots. Additional sources: Meat, Eggs, Cheese, Milk, Spinach, Broccoli and Cabbage

Vitamin B

The B vitamins keep strands strong and plentiful. They assist in maintaining the strength of the hair.

Vitamin B3 (Niacin)

Niacin aids in blood flow and circulation to the scalp, which brings more blood to the source of the hair. Niacin also helps to flush out *dihydrotestosterone*, or DHT, the active form of the male hormone that contributes to Male Pattern Baldness.

Vitamin B5 (Pantothenic Acid)

Pantothenic Acid is a popular ingredient in hair products. It leaves the hair shiny and makes the hair more absorbent to moisture.

Vitamin B6 and B12

The primary role of Vitamins B6 and B12 is to create melanin, which gives hair its color. An absence of either of these vitamins will lead to premature greying.

Vitamin B9 (Folic Acid)

Folic acid not only helps your hair grow faster, it also aids in attaining healthier hair. Because it operates at the level of cell division, Folic Acid helps the hair to reproduce strong resilient strands from the follicles to the hair ends, which has a positive impact on the health, look and feel of your hair. *Food Source for Vitamin B: Chicken, Turkey, Fish, Brewer's Yeast, Whole Grain, Eggs and Milk*

Vitamin C

Vitamin C helps to prevent hair loss, dryness, brittle hair and split ends. It is an antioxidant for hair health. Vitamin C helps to fight the bacteria on the scalp. It wards off dandruff, helps to get rid of the follicles' debris and encourages new hair to grow. Vitamin C also aids dry and itchy scalps because of its anti-viral properties. It also helps the body to form collagen which keeps the skin firm and youthful.

Food Source: Citrus Fruits, Potatoes and Dark Green Vegetables

Vitamin D

Vitamin D helps to provide nourishment for the hair follicles and works in conjunction with protein to form strong hair.

Food Source: Dairy products, Greek yogurt, Cottage Cheese, Low Fat Cheese and Milk

Vitamin E

Vitamin E is an antioxidant that enhances blood circulation to the scalp and promotes new blood vessels. It helps to protect hair from free radicals and helps hair to retain moisture. Vitamin E is not only good internally; it is a great topical agent for hair. As a topical agent, Vitamin E adds moisture to hair and helps hair to maintain its luster delivered by coloring agents.

Food source: Nuts, Leafy Green Vegetables, Beans and Wheat Germ Oil

Other Nutrients and Factors

Fiber

Elimination is another important aspect of a healthy hair diet. Once you have consumed all of the good nutrients, it is important to eliminate waste regularly. When food stays in our bodies too long it ferments, and increases the amount of bacteria and toxins in the body; which inhibits the absorption of nutrients in the bloodstream. A fiber-rich diet helps the body to discard the inhibitors.

Food source: Bran, Cauliflower, Leafy Green Vegetables, Celery, Squash and Beans

Water

Once you've consumed good nutrients, drinking plenty of water is crucial. Water helps absorption of vitamins and nutrients into the blood stream. After absorption, water helps the nutrients move through the blood to the hair and scalp, and rids the body of toxins.

Did you know that 25% of your hair is composed of water? Water is what makes hair moist and gives it elasticity and sheen. Water also helps the body to eliminate any toxins that would harmful to the body or impede hair growth. Although it is not always a cure, most dandruff and flaky scalp conditions will improve dramatically with an increase of water intake.

Smoking and Sleep

Either smoking or not getting enough sleep can affect how your hair looks and feels. No magic nutrient can make up for these practices. However, if your diet is lacking any of the vitamins and nutrients we discussed, or if your body is not processing any of these nutrients as it should, a good multivitamin is recommended to fill in the gaps and give you the proper nutrition necessary for hair growth.

Note: The food source listed after each nutrient is not conclusive and should be used only as a guide. ♥~CF

Products

As a veteran stylist, I am still overwhelmed when I enter a beauty supply store. So many pretty bottles and smell good products, all promising to be the magic bullet for luxurious hair. How is the average consumer supposed to choose?

Please know that any product promising dramatic hair growth is pulling your leg. Hair grows about ½-inch month, and products can be used to both sustain the growth and protect against environmental factors. Although a lot of revolutionary products are out there on the market, it is important to use products that are specific to your individual hair care needs. Even a *good* product can be detrimental if not *properly* used.

Let's talk a look at some of the more common products and talk about how to choose them and use them.

Shampoos

The primary purpose of shampoo is to cleanse the hair and scalp to maintain proper hair and scalp hygiene. It is also the foundation of any service that requires heat. Dirty hair is three times more likely to burn. To be effective a shampoo must remove all oils, dirt and debris without adversely affecting the scalp or the integrity of the hair.

Oily Hair/ Balancing Shampoos remove the excess oils and hydrate both the hair and scalp. The ultimate goal for all hair is to find a moisture balance. Tipping the scales in either direction presents its challenges. The occurrence of oily hair is due to overactive sebaceous or oil-making glands.

Moisturizing Shampoos seek to add moisture to the hair. Dry hair is often the result of under-active sebaceous glands or from other damage to the hair. Shampoos with strong detergents, chemically processing the hair, heating tools and even environmental factors can cause such damage.

Moisturizing shampoos are designed to make the hair smooth and shiny, avoid any further damage and improve manageability. They are typically fortified with conditioners that restore both moisture and elasticity. Shampoo alone is usually not enough to balance the moisture, but it's a great building block.

Clarifying Shampoos are acidic and formulated to cut through product buildup, which will increase shine. It's important to note that you should only use clarifying shampoo when needed because they can be rough on your hair. You should definitely avoid clarifying shampoos after getting your hair colored. Even the mildest clarifying shampoos will remove some of the color.

Color-Treated Shampoos are used to enhance color, gently add a hint of color or remove unwanted color tones. Color-treated shampoos are especially popular for persons with grey, blonde or red hair. These shampoos combine the use of cleansing surfactants with basic color pigments. They are similar to temporary color rinses because they are translucent and can be washed out easily.

Acid Balanced/ pH Balanced Shampoos have a pH that matches that of the skin; 4.5 to 5.5. These shampoos are designed to close the cuticle so they are highly recommended after a chemical service.

Neutralizing Shampoos are **Acid Balanced Shampoos**. They have a pH of 4.5 to 5.5. They are to be used after a chemical relaxer, and designed to remove the relaxer from the hair and return hair to a normal pH. Neutralizing shampoos must be used after a relaxer because relaxers are highly alkaline and water alone does not neutralize the hair.

Volumizing Shampoos are designed to cleanse thoroughly thin, limp or fine hair. These shampoos aid in removing the excess oils and debris which makes it difficult for hair to stand. Volumizing shampoos should be lightweight and rinse off well. Some of them are even fortified with a product to swell the hair shaft so it can appear more buoyant. Some caution should be used when picking a volumizing shampoo to ensure you don't cause any damage to already fine, limp hair. Make certain to use a lightweight conditioner that rinses off well so you don't reverse the benefits of the shampoo.

Dandruff/ Medicated Shampoos contain special medicines or minerals, often Zinc, which relieves excessive dandruff or other conditions of the scalp. To be effective, the shampoo should rest on the scalp for a period of time. Follow manufacturer's recommendations. These special shampoos are usually drying to the hair and should be followed by a conditioning agent. Caution should be exercised when using on color treated hair because the harshness of these shampoos often removes some of the color.

Dry/ Powder Shampoos use a powder to pick up dirt and oils while brushing the hair, without any water. Dry shampoos are usually reserved for clients who physically cannot manage a wet shampoo due to the pressure of the shampoo bowl or shower. However, they have gained some popularity as a good way to refresh the hair without a full shower and blow-dry. Dry shampoo or powder is an effective way to remove oil from excessively oily hair.

Sulfate Free Shampoos offer a milder or gentler alternative for cleansing hair. Most shampoos use a detergents or surfactant known as sodium lauryl sulfate, or SLS. The SLS makes the products sudsy and helps to cleanse the hair. Although the surfactants are often balanced with moisturizers, they can still be harsh and drying and can cause color to fade prematurely. Sulfate Free Shampoos cleanse by using natural antibacterial agents.

Conditioners

Leave-in conditioners are applied to the hair and not rinsed out. They are low in pH and are used to balance the hair after a chemical service or even swimming, both of which can elevate the pH of hair. Leave-in conditioners are often used to detangle hair and add moisture. Leave-ins do not rely on heavy oils; instead, they incorporate lighter, water soluble moisturizers including glycerin and panthenol. Good on most hair types, these conditioners are best for reducing frizz and serve as a thermal (heat) protectant.

Instant conditioners are considered instant because of their short application time; usually one to five. They are water based and contain humectants to improve dry and brittle hair. They will often possess heat-protecting agents to reduce damage and breakage to the hair caused by heated styling tools. People with minimal dryness or fine hair may find instant conditioners a better solution than the heavier moisturizing conditioners. An instant conditioner can also be used as a maintenance conditioner.

Moisturizers are heavier than instant conditioners and require a longer application time, usually 10 to 20 minutes. Often moisturizers use the same ingredients as instant conditioners, but they are in heavier concentration, and formulated to penetrate deep within the strand and to have a longer staying power. Because of the weight of these moisturizers, they are recommended for medium to coarse textured hair, and hair that is brittle, breaks easily and lacks elasticity.

Note: The over use of moisturizers will cause hair to feel heavy, too soft and evens causes tangling.

Protein conditioners are used to improve the strength of the hair, add volume and temporarily close split ends. Keratin is often lost from the hair through chemical treatments and over exposure to heat. Concentrated protein (liquid) is designed to pass through the cuticle, strengthen the cortex (inner layer of hair), equalize porosity and increase elasticity. Protein conditioners are good for hair that feels spongy, limp and overly soft.

Note: Proteins require caution because while they strengthen hair, when used too often they result is improper moisture balance. Important to note is the fact that a protein imbalance is often followed by a moisture loss of some degree. Proteins are meant to add structure, but too much structure makes the hair rigid and decreases its elasticity.

Reconstructing conditioners and hair masks are deep penetrating conditioners that combine a concentrated protein in the heavy cream base of a moisturizer. They penetrate the cuticle layer and are the chosen therapy when both moisturizers and proteins are needed.

Note: Reconstructing conditioners vary in the balance of moisture and protein. As a result, they vary in effectiveness for each individual.

Hot oil treatments are used to prevent dry scalp, minimize damage from harmful styling practices such as heated tools and color, and prevent frizz. When hair is extremely porous and hard to hold moisture, hot oil treatments are suggested to lock in moisture.

Note: Remember, natural, plant-based oils work best to provide nourishment for the hair as opposed to weighting it down and clogging pores with petroleum or mineral-based oils. Plant-based oils include almond, argan, camellia, grape seed and olive.

Oils and Serums both add shine to hair and act as a heat protectant for the hair. Most hair oils are natural, meaning extracted from plants, and is used to penetrate the hair and add moisture. Oils will usually soften and smooth the cuticle and serums will seal the cuticle. Serums are silicon-based and tend to be lightweight, making it a good product for all hair types. Because serums seal the cuticle, some caution should be taken when using serums on dry hair because it can seal the cuticle and thus make it difficult for moisture to penetrate the hair shaft.

Setting lotions are designed to be used on wet hair during the setting process. They contribute to ease in setting, molding and defining the hair, and are purposed to add body to a style. Setting lotions usually come in a concentrated form and can be diluted to yield a soft, medium or firm hold. They are good for all hair types, yet the amount of hold necessary is determined by the hair type.

Gels and Pomades are both used to add texture, mold the hair and make the hair manageable. Gels are usually applied to wet hair to mold hair for a managed set or for a definitive style. Gels come in various holds to suit different hair types and textures. Pomades are wax-based products used on dry hair. They are also used for styling short hair. Pomades also have some hold, but offer a less defined look. With any product, use modestly because excessive amounts can cause the hair to be weighed down and even flaky. In the case of pomade, using too much will make the hair look greasy.

Hairspray and oil sheens are both applied to the hair either by mist or aerosol sprays. The hairspray or finishing spray can be applied before styling the hair, but is usually applied to a finished look to hold the hair in place. Finishing sprays come in variety of strengths. The one you choose depends on the level of hold you want and your hair type.

Note: The firmness of the hold is usually is an indication of higher alcohol contents, which in turn can dry the hair. Oil sheens are also applied to a finished look, but they are not designed to hold the hair. Instead, oil sheens are designed to add a shiny finish to the look. Oil sheens help to reflect the natural sheen of hair. **Although they have oil contents, oil sheens are not designed to penetrate the hair shaft and add moisture. Apply oil sheen sparingly, because excessive amounts can weigh the hair down, causing it to be limp and appear greasy.**

With time, patience and much attentiveness, you will learn to balance your individual hair care needs. When applying products remember to start with a little and add more as needed. Too much of any good thing can pose a problem. Whenever possible, emulsify products in your hands before applying them to the hair. Using this method will help to avoid over-saturation of products in a particular area.

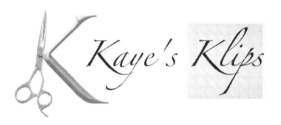

When applying product to the hair, always emulsify the product in the hands to distribute it more evenly and to avoid clumping. Always start applying products in the back of the head and work towards the top to avoid over saturation.

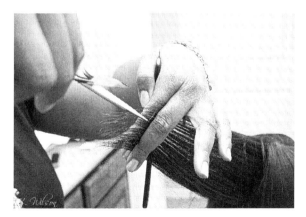

Routine Maintenance

Like most things in life, hair requires tender loving care and gentle treatment to maintain its luster. Hair is subject to many extremes; from the winter winds and summer heat to pollutants, dirt, chemicals and heated tools.

TLC is a must in hair maintenance. Use this list of maintenance tips to keep your mane tame:

♥Shampoo and condition often. Dirty hair is three times more likely to burn. Once you shampoo your hair, seal it with conditioner to lock in the moisture.

♥Conduct due diligence to find a product specific for your hair type.

♥Ensure hair is wet thoroughly before applying shampoo. Doing this helps to minimize breakage or tangling.

♥Apply shampoos mostly to the scalp where oils and debris accumulate. Apply conditioners mostly to the hair ends that are more prone to dryness.

♥Avoid combing or brushing wet hair.

♥Remove all tangles and snarls before shampooing to avoid excessive tangling.

♥Avoid roughing or pulling the hair while shampooing. Be gentle when shampooing; hair is most fragile when wet.

♥Minimize use of clarifying and dandruff shampoos for hair that tangles easily. They will often intensify the tangling.

♥Refrain from use of *hot* water; it will strip the hair of its natural oils causing it to be dry and brittle.

♥Wash combs, brushes, pillowcases and all scarves or head wraps weekly to ensure cleanliness of hair.

♥Protect your hair. Heated tools deliver great looks, but they can also burn hair. Use caution when using heated tools.

Many environmental factors adversely affect the hair. Use these tips to protect your hair:

♥Air-dry whenever possible to limit exposure heated tools.

♥Thoroughly towel-dry your hair before blow-drying. Dry the hair at 70% before using a brush.

♥Avoid using the hottest dryer or even the hottest setting on the blow dryer, especially when the service will be followed with another heated tool.

♥Point the blow dryer down on the hair shaft when blow drying to avoid frizz in the hair.

♥Don't leave the blow dryer or any heated tools in one area of your hair too long. Doing so can cause the hair to burn and break.

♥Add products with sunblock to hair before extreme sun exposure.

♥Use serum to repel static or tame frizz and flyaway hair strands.

♥To minimize sun exposure; consider wearing a hat when planning a prolonged stay in the sun.

♥Use a *satin* pillowcase or scarf. Satin helps to maintain the hair's moisture; cotton absorbs moisture making the hair dryer.

Use these tips when styling your hair:

♥Lightly mist your finished style with a hairspray to hold the look in place.

♥Refrain from the temptation of applying chemicals too often.

♥Extend the time between chemical services to about eight weeks.

♥When brushing longer hair, brush the ends first to remove tangles. Then move up the hair shaft until you can take full strokes from the scalp to the hair ends.

♥Use a leave-in conditioner before styling hair. It will balance the pH, help keep hair hydrated, act as a heat protectant and keep the hair tangle free.

♥A ponytail is a great style to reduce heat and excessive styling.

♥When pulling your hair up, avoid pulling hair too tight. Excessive pulling can cause breakage.

♥Exercise caution when using products with high alcohol content because they are drying to the hair.

Remember these tips when cutting your hair:
♥Trim regularly. The ends of your hair split as they age. Get a trim on average every eight to 10 weeks.
♥Leave cutting to the experts as much as is possible.
♥Never use a dull razor on a cut or trim; doing so will leave ends frayed and hair frizzy.
♥Exercise caution when texturizing hair with shears. Too much texturizing or thinning will leave the hair frizzy.

Trends are ever changing, but a constant, universal trend is healthy hair. What good is it to make the investment in designer shoes and clothes, yet fail miserably when it comes to *the mane attraction*? The conditioning treatments and products available today can help restore damaged hair. Even so, protect the hair from damage whenever possible, because an ounce of prevention beats a pound of cure!

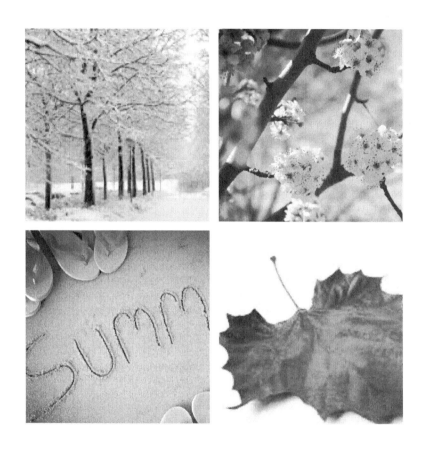

Chapter III
Best Tressed for Every Season

Life is all about seasons. To everything there is a season. When we hear the word *seasons* we automatically think of the four seasons of the year; but a season is marked by a period of time. As you progress through the seasons of your life, your hair care needs change and it is important to change your regimen to accommodate those changing needs.

Let's take a look at some of the seasons of life, and the challenges that are often faced during that time so you can be well prepared. I'd like to offer some hair tips to help you to navigate through those seasons of life. Hot or cold, young or old, use these tips to stay in step and maintain beautiful tresses all year, every year, every season.

Infant Hair Care

It all starts here. Even when babies are born with a head full of thick hair, it often falls out within a few months. One of the reasons babies' hair falls out is because their little bodies are stabilizing in development. At birth, babies' hormones levels are high from their mother. Shortly after birth, when hormone levels decrease, many hair strands go into the telogen or resting phase. When this happens the hair falls out and the hair growth cycle begins. If your baby is bald, there is no reason for alarm. If the baby is two or older and still experiences no hair growth, confer with your pediatrician.

Here are a few tips to manage baby hair:

♥**Understand Cradle Cap.** A common concern for new mothers, Cradle Cap is the name given to the yellowish or white scales that appear on a baby's scalp within the first few months. The exact cause for cradle cap is unknown, but the most common theory is that it is a form of dandruff and is caused by the sebaceous glands. Whatever the cause, what is known is the scales are not contagious, and they do not cause any pain or discomfort to the child.

To treat Cradle Cap shampoo often; keep the scalp oiled with olive oil or Vaseline® and brush gently with a baby brush to loosen the scales. Be careful not to pick the scales; doing so can irritate the child's scalp.

♥**Resist hair ornaments.** Although the temptation is great to adorn little girls with beautiful bows and headbands, be careful. A baby's hair is so fine; the bows can be heavy and cause breakage. A greater danger is the risk of the bow or headband falling off and posing a choking hazard.

♥**Manage baby's bald spots.** Babies' hair often dries out because they are lying on and always rubbing against cotton blankets that absorb all moisture. Babies also tend to lie in the same spot, which causes friction and makes the hair rub off. No worries! The hair will grow back when they start to sit up more so there is no need to concern yourself with harsh products.

♥**Avoid the temptation to pull the hair tight** for cornrows or ponytails. This is painful for babies and can lead to alopecia.

♥**Avoid putting pressure on the soft spot** on the top of the baby's head. This is not necessarily bad for the hair, rather for the child's overall well-being.

Child's Play - Hair Care for Children

Children have endless hours of perspiring, running, jumping and playing in the sandbox. Endless exposure to sun, humidity and other environmental pollutants tend to be drying to those precious locks.

Here are some recommendations that will manage hair care for your children:

♥**Shampoo weekly.** The endless fun of a child can lead to nightmares for parents. Lice and the fungus that causes *tinea capitis*, popularly known as ringworm, are often lurking in the sandbox. Shampoo your child's hair regularly to avoid such dangers.

♥**Use Moisturizing shampoos and conditioners** often. Perspiration is drying to the hair and the constant exposure to the elements depletes hair of its moisture.

♥**Start trimming routinely** as a part of the maintenance process. All of the rubbing, pulling and horse playing causes friction in the hair and roughens up the hair shaft. Trimming regularly helps to keep hair looking smooth.

♥**Brace yourself!** Playing fantasy beauty salon is all in child's play. Often I see little ones in the salon that have chopped off their bang, or even a ponytail. While, I find it hilarious and see it as an indicator of a bold, creative mind; most parents are mortified by the event.

Watch children carefully when scissors are near, but brace yourself for their first real haircut. If this happens, take them to a stylist accustomed to working with children. If the cut is really severe, keep in mind a healthy child's hair will grow back quickly – and the stores carry cute hats for children!

♥**Avoid Harsh Chemicals.** Although adorning our little ones with the latest fashion trends and styles is always exciting, avoid the temptation to apply harsh chemicals such as perms, chemical relaxers and colors. Such chemicals require upkeep which can be a daunting task; in addition they can cause irritation to sensitive, youthful skin.

♥**Lookout for *tinea capitis*, or Ringworm,** a fungi that appears on the scalp and is common in children. It appears on the scalp as a bald patch of scaly skin, or on the skin in a ring shaped rash. Fungi grow well in warm moist places.

Ringworms are characterized by itching, hair loss in the form of round dry patches, pus, swelling and in some cases fever. Ringworm should not be treated by a hair care specialist or random home remedies. Schedule a visit with a physician at the onset because the longer ringworm goes untreated the worse it becomes.

Until you see a physician, keep skin clean and dry. Change sheets often. Caution should be used when handling ringworm because it can spread throughout the head or even be passed from person to person.

♥**Lice** are another concern in hair care for children. Head lice are parasites; insects that feed off the scalp and can be transferred from person to person. Lice are found most often in children between the ages of three to 11 and in persons living in the household with an infested child. Lice are very rarely found in African Americans because their hair texture makes it more difficult for the louse to survive.

The Centers for Disease Control (CDC) recommends that any person with active lice see a physician, but there are some non-prescription medications that are effective. Visit www.cdc.gov/parasites/lice for more information on lice and over the counter medication recommendations.[5]

Note: The CDC also warns: Do not use a combination shampoo and conditioner, or conditioner before using lice medicine. Do not re-wash the hair for 1-2 days after the lice medicine is removed.

Puberty

If your child is experiencing hair growth in new areas, growth spurts, body odor, developing breasts in girls, or getting a deep voice in boys then welcome to puberty! If you can remember puberty and recall it to be a perplexing time for you, know that it comes with the same perplexities for your child.

With the influx of hormones come a lot of changes. One of the biggest changes is over active sebaceous glands.

The following cautions will help to manage hair care for preteens and balance oil production:

♥**Use anti-fungal or dandruff shampoo.** Hormone imbalance and over active sebaceous glands are common triggers for dandruff. When acne is present in pre-teens, most often it is accompanied by dandruff. The use of an anti-fungal shampoo *(zinc pyrithione or selenium zinc)* will help to slow down skin cell production.

♥**Don't over shampoo.** Shampooing the hair regularly is a part of routine hygiene, but using too many shampoos or shampooing too often stimulates the already active sebaceous glands and the result is excessively oily hair.

♥**Go green.** A diet rich in leafy green vegetables and fruit is good to boost hair growth and flush out toxins from the over-active sebaceous glands. By contrast, a diet that favors too much refined sugar and cereals triggers dandruff and excessive oil production.

♥**Use mild shampoos.** While hormones are balancing, it is important to help the hair maintain its pH. Harsh shampoos or more alkaline shampoos will irritate the scalp. You should know that the softer a shampoo, the less it will foam and the less it risks aggravating your sebaceous glands.

♥**Avoid using the hairdryer at high temperatures.** Using the blow dryer on high temperatures and placing it too close to the scalp will artificially dry out the skin and scalp, and proportionally stimulate the secretion of sebum.

Experimenting with Hair In Your 20's

Experimentation, exploration and self-discovery are good terms to describe life in your 20's. This is a transitional season, and most women are beginning to come into their own sense of self. In doing so, they tell their story with their hair. Hair often endures much abuse during this period.

Here are some clues to help you brave these new hair adventures:

♥**Develop good hair habits**. Developing good hair practices now will definitely pay off in the long run.

♥**Use heat protectants.** While experimenting with all the new looks, ensure to protect the hair from excessive heating tools. Styling devices can reach temperatures up to 450°F and cause micro-fine damage to wet, unprotected hair. The long-term consequences are split ends and breakage. Most hair care companies feature products designed to protect the hair from heat; they range from shampoos and conditioners, to wet sprays to be applied during the drying process, and oils and serums.

♥**Massaging your scalp** for a few minutes each day will stimulate circulation which makes the scalp more supple, stimulate the blood flow towards the roots, and boost hair growth. Massaging the scalp also helps to prevent dandruff. When massaging your scalp be careful not to tangle the hair and cause breakage. The relaxation that comes from the massage is an added bonus.

♥**Exercise caution with chemical services.** Each new style or fad is often accompanied by a new chemical: Colors, straighteners, relaxers or permanent waves. Even so, be careful not to apply them too often and over process the hair, leaving it fragile and brittle.

♥**Beware of postnatal hair loss.** The 20's is a time when most women start having children. Though your hair may grow and seem extra full during pregnancy, experiencing shedding shortly after giving birth is not uncommon. Because of the excessive amounts of hormones present during pregnancy, hair does not shed as a part of the hair growth cycle. After child birth there is a dramatic decline of the hormones and all of the hair that would have shed normally during pregnancy sheds at once. Although this experience is often a vexation, don't panic. The hair will resume the natural hair growth cycle and return to the anagen, or growing phase with proper maintenance and a healthy diet.

♥Look at hormonal imbalances in birth control pills. Some birth control pills are high in estrogen, which tends to promote hair growth; while others are high in progesterone, which encourages hair loss. It is important to have your physician monitor your hormonal levels while on the pill to ensure your hormones are in balance,

♥Avoid fad diets. As discussed in Chapter II, a healthy and balanced diet is vital to hair health. Diets that eliminate entire food groups can cause you to abandon nutrients that are critical for hair health. If your diet is lacking specific nutrients, a good multi-vitamin should be a supplement.

Hair In Your 30's

Life in your 30's is about adjusting to all of the changes you have embraced in the last decade. Balancing the needs of marriage, children, careers and anything else you have taken on can be a daunting task.

The following insider information should help you make the necessary adjustments:

♥De-stress. You have a lot on your plate. Find an outlet to alleviate stress, because chronic stress can cause physiological changes in the body which can lead to hair loss.

♥Check your iron. This is a time when many women will start to experience a heavier menstrual flow. The increased blood loss often leads to low iron. This decrease in iron can lead to hair loss. Even slight anemia may often lead to thinning of the hair.

♥Soften it up. Hard, stiff hairstyles require hairspray or gel. Hairspray and gels use a lot of alcohol which dries the hair out. Very dry, brittle hair is prone to breakage.

♥Let it shine. Maintain your youthful looking locks with lots of natural shine. To keep your hair looking shiny and vibrant, get a color gloss. A color gloss refreshes your hair color, seals the ends for a healthier look and adds tons of light-reflecting shine. Avoid mousses and aerosol sprays that leave a matte finish on the hair. Instead, opt for serums and shine sprays – but use them modestly to avoid looking greasy.

Taming Hair In Your 40's (Pre-Menopause)

By the time you reach your 40's you have had enough life experiences to be self-assured and confident. You are at the top of your game, so don't let your hair stop the show! If your hair is a problem, fix it.

The following tips will equip you to face some of your hair challenges in your 40's:

♥Keep it current. With all of your new responsibilities it's easy to get stuck in a rut. Don't get too comfortable with an 'easy' hairstyle and fail to embrace change. Nothing dates your look like wearing an outdated hairstyle. Your stylist can help you find a look that will fit your hair type and texture, and also be suitable for your lifestyle.

♥**Be gentle.** As you age your hair becomes more fragile. Only use a wide-toothed comb when combing wet hair and always use a soft bristle brush. Don't comb aggressively. Handle your hair like you would a delicate fabric.

♥**Look at the grey area.** Most women will start to see some greying in their 40's. Now is the time to look at the grey and determine if you will color or if you will prepare for the silver screen. Wearing grey is an option that suites some, but know that wearing grey requires a lot of maintenance. Either way, treat the grey to keep it shiny or to eliminate it.

♥**Turn down the heat.** Many women in their 40's have already noticed their hair to be thinner than it was in their 20's. Because there is less density, less heat is required. Use less heat with your heated tools to avoid burning your hair.

Maintaining Hair in Your 50's and Beyond

Does life begin at 40, 50 or 60? We are living better and all of our former benchmarks seem to be shifting. Along with our benchmarks, in your 50's many things in your body will also be shifting. Menopause is a major transformation that takes place in women during this time. When your hormones shift, adjusting your beauty regime to accommodate this change is crucial. By making the following adjustments you will be prepared for the refinement:

♥**Get your thyroid checked.** In her book *Hormone Harmony*, Jill Waggoner, M.D. discusses hypothyroidism, which occurs when the body does not produce enough of the thyroid hormone. Hypothyroidism is a disease that often affects menopausal women. Symptoms of this disorder include obesity and heart disease, but it can also result in a thinner head of hair. If you notice your hair thinning, consider having your doctor to perform a thyroid function test to see if you are experiencing optimal performance.

♥**Learn to camouflage thinning hair.** As you get older the hair growth cycle slows down, it takes longer to grow hair and the hair strands get thinner. Remember these tips to help disguise thinning hair:

> ♥Add layers; this makes hair look fuller.
>
> ♥Get multi-dimensional color. Highlights and lowlights add dimension to a style and make the hair look fuller.

♥Add curls. Curls make it more difficult to see through hair and makes hair look fuller.

♥Avoid long styles that lay flat to this head. This draws attention to thinning hair.

♥Make it orange. As you mature, the body produces less moisture. As a result, your hair and skin tends to lack moisture. The orange foods are rich in beta-carotene. Beta-carotene is not a nutrient, but it is a precursor of vitamin A. The body converts beta-carotene to vitamin A, which will help you to produce more sebum (the fluid produced by the body to keep the hair and skin moisturized).

♥Deep condition regularly. Because your body tends to produce less moisture over time, dry hair becomes more evident. Increasing your water intake is always a good idea, but deep conditioners will also help to deflect the lack of moisture.

♥Don't pull it out! Life, menopause and the symptoms thereof can make you feel crazy. Your challenge is to stay calm, no matter how overwhelming life may seem. Be careful not to pull all of your hair out!

Winter Hair

The most wonderful time of the year has to be Winter. Love is in the air, while the fireplaces are roaring: Families are bonding and old Saint Nick is making his list and checking it twice. Winter with all its splendor can wreak havoc on your hair. From the extremes of the biting winds and bitter cold outside to the overheated furnace inside, the moisture in your hair doesn't stand a chance.

Consider these Do's and Don'ts to gear up for Jack Frost:

1. **DO add a moisture intense conditioning mask to your regimen.** This will help the hair to stay moist and handle the super drying conditions of "Old Man Winter."

2. **DO increase your intake Vitamins B5, C and E.** These vitamins help the hair to retain moisture.

3. **DON'T forget the humidifier.** Because the air is so dry inside and outside in the winter, adding a humidifier to your home will help replace the moisture in the air. Not only will it be great for your hair, your skin, nails and nasal passages will also benefit.

4. **DO use oil, moisturizing lotion or a serum.** These moisturizers applied lightly will help to de-frizz "hat" hair

and static. They will also act as a shield to protect your hair from the brutal winter winds and add shine.

5. **DON'T use heated tools on dry hair.** Heated tools affect moisture-starved hair more than usual, leaving it dull and brittle and it increases breakage.

Winter usually means dry, dry, dry. With these helpful tips, dry isn't in the forecast for your hair!

Spring Hair

My thoughts for the Spring are always bittersweet. Spring brings April showers and budding flowers. Everything is growing, including your hair. Hair grows more in Spring and Summer than in Fall and Winter. Although the budding flowers are a beautiful and welcomed sight after Winter's cold, the budding flowers also mean allergies, allergies, allergies! The result is taking lots of allergy medicines, which are designed to dry up a nasal drip. The unfortunate side effect of these medicines is that they dry out the hair and skin.

At onset of Spring we move from the harsh dry Winter to a moist, humid time of year. The biggest challenge is to balance the hair's moisture.

Consider these Do's and Don'ts to help your hair Spring forward:

1. **DO trim your ends.** Because Winter can be so harsh on your hair, it's a good idea to start with a trim to keep it looking neat and tame.

2. **DO drink plenty of water.** If you are taking antihistamines, it is important to replenish the body of its moisture. Also, all growth needs water to sustain it. Water your roots.

3. **DON'T forget to swap conditioners.** Winter is extremely drying, and the hair needs intense moisture. You will still need to deep condition, but maybe not as much. The spring humidity combined with excessive moisturizers will make your hair hard to manage. Swap for a lighter conditioner.

4. **DO shampoo regularly.** If you are using an antihistamine it is a good idea to shampoo at least once a week with a clarifying shampoo to remove the medicine build-up.

5. **DO refresh color.** Spring is a colorful time of the year. The days look brighter and so should your hair. Start with a refreshing color for the spring. This helps to give the

hair a lustrous shiny finish and helps you to look slightly kissed by the sun.

6. **DON'T forget your accessories**. Hair ornaments are always a plus, but Spring is a perfect time to add a flower. Pick a flower and stick it in your hair. You will be right in step with nature.

Spring represents all of nature's pretty blooms. Put some spring into your strands so your hair can reflect the splendor of the season.

Summer Hair

From backyard barbecues, to family reunions and a weekend at the beach; there is always a "sun-thing" to do. Sun exposure is drying and damaging to the hair. Too much sun exposure often leaves your tresses brittle, frizzy and with ragged ends. Consider these Do's and Don'ts to maintain your summer mane:

1. **DO protect your hair from heat.** An ounce of prevention beats a pound of cure! Use products like serums or leave-in conditioners that have SPF or heat protectants. Wear styles that don't require as much heat such as braids, roller sets and ponytails. When directly in the sun, wear hats or protective gear when possible.

2. **DON'T over-style.** To help protect the hair from drying, let your hair dry naturally as often as possible. Only blow dry or use heated tools when necessary. This will help to protect your hair from additional heat exposure.

3. **DO moisturize your hair.** Lavish your hair with moisturizing shampoos and deep penetrating moisturizing conditioners. These products help to replenish the moisture lost in the sun.

4. **DO pre-treat the hair with leave-in conditioner before swimming.** When the hair is dry and you go swimming, the hair absorbs all of the chlorinated water. By slightly misting the hair with leave-in conditioner the hair absorbs the conditioner and like a sponge, it doesn't have much room to absorb the chlorine.

5. **DO shampoo after each swim.** Swimming is a great past time for the heat, but the chlorine from the pool or salt water from the beach can be extremely harsh and drying to your hair. Always shampoo with a balancing shampoo after every swim.

6. **DO drink plenty of water.** It is always important to drink water, but hydration is crucial for both your physical and hair health when dealing with Summer's heat. I can't say it too much: Hydrate, hydrate, hydrate!

Summer should be the most carefree time of the year. The long days and short nights symbolize fun. Have fun with your hair!

Fall

In the fall, leaves begin to drop from the trees. As it is in nature, so it is with you. Hair begins to shed more in the Fall. Although normal shedding is about 50 to 100 strands daily, during Fall it is not uncommon to see it double to as many as 150 to 200 strands daily. If shedding is more aggressive or lasts longer than two-three weeks, it could indicate there is a more serious problem.

Consider these Do's and Don'ts to keep your hair on the fashion forecast for Fall:

1. **DO use a leave in conditioner after each shampoo.** This will help to replenish nutrients lost during this period.
2. **DO increase protein in your diet.** When hair start to shed, a protein rich diet helps to strengthen hair fibers.
3. **DO monitor chemical service while hair is shedding excessively.** If the hair is shedding you want to be extremely careful about introducing service that might compromise the integrity of your hair.

4. **Do freshen up color for the fall.** The colors of Fall are rich, so why not join in with nature? When you start to spend less time in the sun, your skin will look lighter. If your hair is not shedding, consider a color to enhance the depth and richness of the hair and make your skin look radiant.

5. **Do keep a shine serum nearby to help fight frizz.** In the Fall you start to wear heavier clothes. These tend to rub the hair and cause more friction. This friction combined with the changing temperature will cause hair to begin experiencing dryness and more frizz. Shine serum will not only give hair a gloss, it will eliminate frizz.

The clock falls back at this time of year, but your hair can fall into fashion and be "best-tressed" in this season!

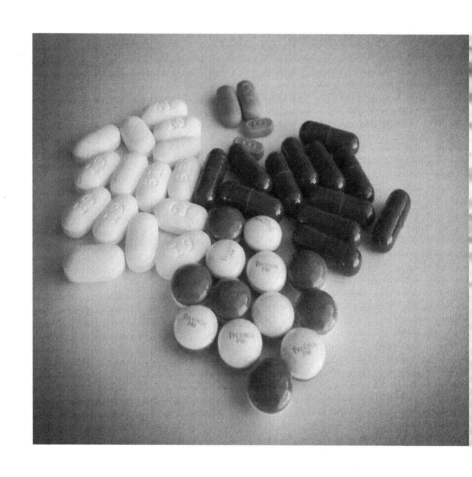

Chapter IV
Medicine Mane

As I stated previously, several years ago I took a medicine and one of the side effect was hair loss. Shortly after that, I read an article listing all of the medications that cause hair loss.[6] I soon learned that many common prescription drugs carry hair loss as a side effect. From the "oh so" common aspirin to beta-blockers, acne to high blood pressure; your medication could be the culprit for hair loss.

Going thin on top? Has your hair texture changed drastically? An alarming amount of medicines have adverse effects on the hair growth cycle. Your doctor may not have mentioned hair loss as a side effect for your prescription. However, conducting your own research is important. Ask your pharmacist for information when you have your prescription filled. A number of websites and medication guidebooks can also serve as additional resources.

Hair loss or thinning can occur up to a year after taking medication but in most cases the hair loss occurs within the first month. When drugs are the cause of hair loss, a few symptoms often accompany the hair loss. Hair feels unusually dry and brittle. The scalp often feels itchy and tender. Medicine induced hair loss is usually diffused throughout the head and the "fallout" appears in long strands from the scalp. Thankfully, in most cases, medicine induced hair loss is reversible.

A number of things that can cause hair loss; medicine is only one of them. If you notice excessive amounts of hair falling out, see your hair care provider so you can take an exhaustive look at possible causes. If you suspect the shedding is as a result of medication, see your physician.

If you are able to determine that your medications are the cause of your hair loss, **do not** try to resolve the issue by discontinuing your medication. Some drugs including prednisone, for example, should never be stopped abruptly; to do so could be harmful. Several medications can be substituted with others that may not cause hair loss as a side effect. Thus, you should always consult with your physician before making any changes to your medications.

The number of medications listing "hair loss" as a side effect is exhaustive. Rather than listing them by name, I will name some of the more common health conditions. Many medicines used to treat these conditions have been found to cause hair loss. The list is not exhaustive; rather it provides a starting point. Call a local pharmacist or consult your physician If you have a question about any medications you are currently taking and their potential to cause hair loss.

Here are some medications listed by categories for common diseases known to cause hair loss:

Acne

Retinoids, which are derived from Vitamin A, are widely used in the treatment of acne. Vitamin A aids in hair growth and sebum production, but because it is fat-soluble it can build up throughout the body; including the hair follicle. Excessive amounts of buildup in the follicle can clog or temporarily shut the follicle down and deter hair growth. The risk increases with the dose and other body hair may be affected as well. If hair loss is a result of excessive amounts of Vitamin A, the hair loss is reversed by reducing the amounts of Vitamin A in the body.

Antidepressants

Among the many drugs known to cause hair loss, antidepressants are one of the most common that frequently results in noticeable thinning. Hair normally sheds at the end of the telogen, or resting phase of the hair growth cycle. Yet with antidepressants, the hair sheds as soon as it enters this phase. However, patients with this problem should not panic. This type of hair loss is reversible and hair growth seems to return rather quickly.

Blood Thinners or High Blood Pressure

Blood thinners, while thinning the blood, often thins the hair. Many years ago, one of the first medications I noticed caused hair loss in my clients was medicines for high blood pressure. I have since learned that any medication that affects the blood; which provides nourishment for the hair, is considered "high risk" for hair loss.

Many clients would complain of tightness of scalp and hair being often drier than normal. Although not limited to the crown, the shedding often appears diffused in the crown area. In some cases, over prolonged use, these medications can cause damage to the hair follicle.

Cholesterol Lowering

Some of your hormones use cholesterol as building blocks; but cholesterol-lowering medicines work to either stop the production of cholesterol in the liver or to block the absorption of cholesterol in the circulatory system. By blocking cholesterol production the hormone balance is affected. By blocking the absorption of cholesterol, these medicines also block the absorption of essential hair growth nutrients.

Contraceptives

In the "high risk" zone for hair loss as a side effect, any drugs directly affecting the hormonal system of the user (birth control pills, steroids, etc.) can cause hair loss. Progesterone based pills are notable for inducing hair loss. *Note: See the section "Hormone Harmony" to understand more on how our hormones effect hair reproduction.*

Diabetes

Although not often discussed, insulin is a peptide hormone that regulates the metabolism of carbohydrates and fats in the body. Any medications that alter the hormones are "high risk" for hair loss.

Epilepsy/Convulsions

Some drugs used for epilepsy and other disorders such as migraines have been linked to hair loss. These drugs may even make hair curly.

Glaucoma

Most glaucoma medicines work to relieve pressure and reduce the production of fluids that build up in the eye. The reduction in fluid production caused by these medicines leads to the hair becoming dry and brittle, thus resulting in breakage.

Inflammation

These groups of medicines are likely the most common as many are sold over the counter. They are used to treat acute to chronic pain and reduce swelling or fever. Hair loss as a result of anti-inflammatory medicines is rare, especially when taken in small doses. However, the risk of hair loss increases with higher doses or prolonged use.

Thyroid disorders

Thyroids are one of the largest of the endocrine glands which secrete hormones. Any medications that alter the hormones are "high risk" for hair loss.

A Word of Caution

If you are taking one or more of these medications and experiencing hair loss, do not take the hair loss as a sign you should quit taking the medication. Before making any adjustments to medications **always** seek advice from your doctor to make sure you are taking the correct dosage and following directions. An alternative medicine that does not cause hair loss may be available.

Be aware of other factors that affect your health and make sure you are taking proper measures such as resting well, exercising, eating a balanced diet and possibly taking a multi-vitamin.

Carefully weigh your options, because although hair loss is definitely painful, hair loss is trivial when you consider the long-term health risk of not taking prescribed medications.

Chemotherapy and Your Hair

A hallmark of cancer is rapid cell reproduction. The goal of chemotherapy is to destroy cancer cells. This is achieved by attacking fast-growing cells. The hair follicle also has rapid cell reproduction. Consequently, as chemotherapy wipes out fast-growing cancer cells, these drugs usually destroy the fast-growing hair cells and inhibit hair growth. Each person with cancer reacts differently to chemotherapy and its various side effects. The severity of hair loss depends primarily on the dosage and type of medicine used in treatment; however nearly all has some degree of hair loss.

Chemotherapy may cause hair loss all over your body — resulting in a form of alopecia known as *alopecia universalis*. Sometimes your eyelash, eyebrow, armpit, pubic and other body hair also falls out. Some chemotherapy drugs are more likely than others to cause alopecia universalis and some range from a mere thinning to complete baldness. During your medical consultation, talk to your physician about what to expect from the medicine you will be taking.

Hair usually begins falling out one to three weeks after you start treatment. It could fall out very quickly in large clumps, or gradually. Significant hair loss is usually noted at 14-21 days into treatment. You'll likely notice accumulations of loose hair on your pillow, in your hairbrush or comb, or in your sink or shower drain. Hair loss is often accompanied by a tender or slightly irritated scalp.

Hair loss will continue throughout the treatment and up to a few weeks afterward. Once the treatment is complete, and the treatment has stopped attacking the cells, hair will slowly re-enter the anagen or growth phase. Initially, the new hair may have a different texture or color than the previous hair; it usually returns to its original texture after a few months.

Several treatments have been investigated as possible ways to prevent hair loss, but none has been proven to be absolute:

Scalp hypothermia / Cold Caps - Tightly fitting skullcaps that are stored on ice or hooked up to a machine (to reach temperatures of 40°F) are applied to the head. As the scalp cools, the blood vessels in the scalp constrict, making it difficult or impossible for the vessels that would otherwise carry the harmful drugs to hair follicles to deliver them. This constriction of blood vessels is also known as *vasoconstriction.* Because the Cold Caps are only applied to the scalp, the "chemo" is then free to work throughout the rest of the body to attack the cancerous cells – while having little to no effect on the scalp.

Studies have found Cold Caps work in the majority of people who have tried it. Many patients report being extremely cold and in some cases the cold is unbearable; headaches and pain in the ears often occurs as the cold sets in. Some patients report that after approximately five minutes into the treatment, the pain goes away after the initial cold shock.

Although the Food and Drug Administration (FDA) has not approved Cold Caps in the United States as medical devices, they are available for rent. Rental fees average $500 monthly.[7]

Minoxidil (Rogaine®) — A drug approved by the FDA for Male Pattern Baldness in men and women that is said to help speed up hair regrowth after treatment. More research is needed to understand whether Minoxidil is effective. However, once the treatment has stopped, a healthy diet helps to promote hair regrowth.

Hair tips for chemotherapy:

Consider cutting your hair prior to treatment.

- o Cutting your hair short before it starts shedding provides a sense of empowerment and the feeling that *you* control when you hair goes short.

- o Short hair tends to look fuller than long hair. As your hair falls out, shedding won't be as noticeable if your hair is short.

- o Cutting your hair short makes the potential transition to total hair loss easier for both you and your family.

Pamper your hair.

- o Get in the habit of being kind to your hair. Pampering your hair now won't prevent "fallout," but it will more likely stay on your head a little longer during treatment.

- o As your hair grows back, remember your hair and scalp is extremely fragile during the first three months. Be gentle in treatment; and don't do any services that you wouldn't do to a child.

o Use a shampoo and conditioner for dry or damaged hair. After treatment, as the hair is growing back, use a gentle sulfate free shampoo.

o Avoid things that will add stress to your hair like tight braids, hair extensions, ponytails, tight elastics, hot rollers or bobby pins. This will also include limiting the use of heated tools.

o When possible simply towel dry. If a hair dryer is needed, keep it on low and several inches from the head.

o Switch to a wide toothed comb and use a soft bristle brush when the hair grows back.

o Avoid styling products that make the hair dry and brittle, i.e., gels, hair sprays and styling mousse.

o Avoid the use of harsh chemicals and permanent colors. For color, use only semi-permanent or demi-permanent colors before, during or immediately following treatment. Go for only subtle color changes. DO NOT USE BLEACH! Bleach or permanent color will not only damage the fragile hair, it will irritate already sensitive scalp and skin.

o Wearing stretch caps or scarves to bed will slow down stress to the hair and catch loose hairs. Waking up to balls of hair on your pillar is very alarming and difficult to process first thing in the morning.

Consider wearing a wig

o Wearing a wig is not mandatory after hair loss, but it often helps make the transition easier. Ask your doctor to write a prescription for a wig; the cost may be covered by your health insurance.

o Sensitivity of the scalp can occur during the falling or shedding phase of the hair. Choosing a wig because of hair loss or medical reasons is different from wearing a wig simply for cosmetic reason. Wigs worn because of medical reasons should be composed of extremely soft and lightweight materials for comfort. Additionally, the use of soft cotton liners during the hair loss-shedding phase will prevent the lost hair from sticking to the inside of the wig cap.

o Although wearing cotton on your hair is usually frowned upon, this is a good time to wear a cotton scarf or liner. It will serve to absorb moisture, keep the head warm and cushion the scalp.

o Protect your scalp if it will be exposed. In direct sunlight, use maximum protection sunscreen or a head covering. In cold weather, use a head covering to insulate your scalp and make you comfortable.

If you are bold enough to go bald, confidence is your best accessory!

Resources:

The **American Cancer Society** is a great resource for helping to deal with the loss of hair, or to steer you in the direction of services available to help you cope. Visit www.cancer.org or call 1.800.227.2345.

Look Good . . . Feel Better is a free program that provides hair and beauty makeovers and tips to women with cancer. These classes are offered throughout the United States and in several other countries. Many classes are offered through local chapters of the American Cancer Society. For more information, visit www.lookgoodfeelbetter.org or call 1.800.395.5665.

Locks of Love is a public non-profit organization that provides hairpieces to financially disadvantaged children under age 18 suffering from medical hair loss. Visit www.locksoflove.org or call 1.888.896.1588 to obtain more information.

Radiation

Radiation therapy also attacks quickly growing cells in your body, but unlike chemotherapy, radiation affects only the specific area where treatment is concentrated. If you have radiation to your head, you will likely lose the hair on your head.

Radiation therapy also affects your skin. The treatment area is likely to be red and may look sunburned or tanned. If your radiation treatment is to your head, it's a good idea when going outside to cover your head with a protective hat or scarf because your skin will be sensitive to cold and sunlight. Wigs and other hairpieces might irritate your scalp.

Hair and Hormones
~by Jill Waggoner, M.D.

Hormone changes and corresponding hair changes are a common problem. Many women experience changes in their hair with the use of contraception, with pregnancy and with menopause.

For most women the most distressful change is hair loss. The hair loss associated with the use of contraceptives is usually temporary and reverses after the contraceptives are stopped. The hair loss that occurs after pregnancy is temporary and levels off after the hormones return to their pre-pregnancy levels. The hair loss that is associated with menopause is usually permanent unless hormone replacement therapy is initiated to alleviate the hormone insufficiency.

So what are hormones and how do they affect the hair?

Hormones are chemical messengers that are secreted by the body's endocrine system which is responsible for most of the major functions in the body. The endocrine system is responsible for regulating metabolism, growth and development, sexual desire, and reproduction. It is composed of a series of glands, for example, the adrenal glands, which release hormones into the bloodstream. These hormones control or regulate various organs and systems of the body.

One hormone in particular, testosterone is one of the reproductive hormones in both men and women; it is responsible for hair loss in both. If testosterone combines with another hormone, *5-alpha reductase* to form an end product called *dihydrotestosterone* (DHT) then hair loss occurs and manifests as pattern baldness in both men and women.

In women the testosterone level increases when estrogen levels decrease or fall. What happens is that DHT attaches itself to cells within those follicles, cells that control normal hair growth. When this attachment occurs, it reduces hair growth during the growing stage and increases the length of time the hair is in the resting stage.

As a result hair is shed at a normal rate but new growth is limited, which means that hair eventually thins and falls out, leading to baldness. If testosterone and DHT are not the problem, other hormones such as estrogen or progesterone could be at fault. One of the most common changes which cause hair loss is experienced during pregnancy. Estrogen levels tend to rise during pregnancy and many women report that their hair has grown longer, thicker and fuller than before. Then suddenly after the birth of their child the hair sheds quickly and dramatically.

Another time of change occurs during menopause. This is the time when a woman's levels of estrogen and progesterone decrease; signaling an end to the reproductive stage of their lives. This change also affects the normal functioning of the hair follicles and disrupts the hair growth.

Because of the increased stimulation of ovaries by the pituitary gland many women produce precursor hormones that can become testosterone. This testosterone increases DHT, and the cascade that is discussed above ensues. As a result new hair growth is delayed or stopped and increased shedding occurs. Thus, the menopausal woman is left with thin hair and some even develop pattern baldness.

Whatever the reason, we understand that it is frustrating or upsetting to lose your hair because of hormonal changes, but help is available. The good news is that most of these hair changes are temporary. Hair growth will return to its regular pattern once the hormone imbalance is corrected, a condition has been treated or the body has returned to its normal state after childbirth.

If however, your hair has not grown after your hormone change has balanced itself or your body is functioning again as normal, then it is time to look at other possibilities as a cause for the problem.[8] *Note: For more information about hormones visit HormoneHarmony4U.com.*

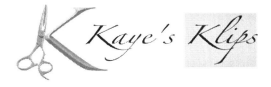

Prior to the 19th century, it was hard to tell a surgeon from a barber or at times a barber from a physician. They all practiced some form of medicine. An interesting aside is the fact that it was medicine's love of the enema that led to surgery becoming a respectable profession.

Previous to 1685, surgeons held little favor with anyone. If you wanted something cut off, you could attend a surgeon or a barber. If you wanted a little bloodletting, you could attend a physician or a barber. Both the surgeon and the barber had that red and white pole outside their place of business.

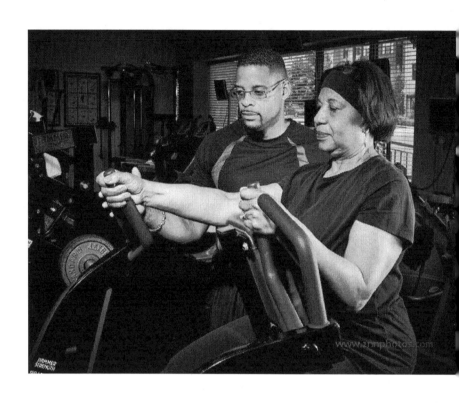

Chapter V
Mane Exercise

It seems almost daily we are bombarded with words and speeches from figures such as Dr. Oz, Dr. Ian Smith, Chris Powell and First Lady Michelle Obama encouraging us to exercise. The benefits of exercise include longevity, weight management, heart health, strength and agility, and overall physical and mental well-being.

Although the warnings against a sedentary lifestyle are heralded daily, we find tons of excuses not to get moving. Amongst those excuses is hair care maintenance. Since taking office, United States Surgeon General Dr. Regina Benjamin encouraged women, and Black women in particular, to go ahead and risk having bad hair days and work out to prevent health disparities like obesity and heart disease. In a quote from the *New York Times*, Dr. Benjamin stated, "Oftentimes you get women saying, 'I can't exercise today because I don't want to sweat my hair back or get my hair wet.'" [9]

I have stated before that I realize a bad hair day often dictates a bad day. For many, starting or ending the day with an exercise regimen means setting aside time to restore *the mane thing.* With the hustle and bustle of a highly automated technological society, this is "extra" time that we often do not have. Besides, who wants to set themselves up for a bad day? I understand our psychological attachments to hair and no one loves a beautiful attractive mane more than me. However, flawless tresses cannot be an excuse to neglect exercise. In fact, healthy and beautiful hair and skin are benefactors of exercise!

A key component in any hair growth or restorative hair plan is increasing the flow of oxygen to the blood stream. Exercise helps you to accomplish that goal. After incorporating a hair healthy diet, exercise is the best way to see the benefits of the dietary regimen.

Hair is nourished by the nutrients circulating through the blood stream. As you exercise, oxygen carries blood to the surface, causing skin to have a nice glow and flushing out toxins that might impede hair growth. Certified Personal Trainer Rod Warner says, "Not only is exercising fun, but nothing helps to get that blood circulating like exercising."

Stress is another impediment to hair growth. Stress is an everyday occurrence for most people. Since it can't be avoided in many cases, managing the body's reaction to stress is very important. Exercise is the vehicle that helps to clear emotional stress from your life. Physical activity will help to manage the normal stress that your body produces as a result of daily activities and unexpected occurrences.

Exercise essentially burns away stress-inducing chemicals like *cortisol* and *norepinephrine*[10]. At the same time, vigorous exercise releases *endorphins*, *dopamine* and *serotonin* into the system. Basically, exercise releases the "feel good" chemicals.

"Exercise is a great way to release pent-up stress. A brisk walk, jogging, swimming, or lifting light weights will help to relieve stress while maintaining a healthy lifestyle," says Warner. "Exercise will help your body process foods and vitamins, sleep better, and reduce stress."

Regular exercise boosts the body's elimination of harmful toxins that impede hair growth. Exercise burns fat, and since most toxins are stored in fat, this helps the body to refuse them. Also, exercise cuts down on the time it takes food to move through the large intestine. This encourages overall well-being and hair health.

Warner says, "I realize some women are afraid of messing their hair up, but that's not the only thing that prohibits us from exercising. Sometimes, they have this preconceived notion that a workout must be strenuous or in a stuffy gym, when in fact it doesn't have to be. There are lots of ways to workout that would be fun, add a sense of adventure and get your heart rate up."

If being in the gym doesn't work for you, Warner offers suggestions for exercising outside of the gym. According to Warner, gardening, dancing, cycling, canoeing, taking nature walks and even jogging present alternate ways for exercising outside of the gym. "The goal is to engage in a nonstop vigorous routine for at least 30 minutes three times a week." Warner continues, "You want to monitor your heart rate, being careful not to exceed the maximum heart rate."

The fitness guru offers these tips for starting an exercise regimen:

Consult a physician. Before beginning any exercise program, consulting with a physician or other qualified health care provider is highly recommended that you. A physician or other health care provider will look at your medical history, any past surgeries and risk factors such as smoking and family history to determine if you are healthy enough for physical activity. This is particularly important if you are:

- Age 40 or over
- Currently inactive
- Significantly overweight
- Someone with a history of heart problems or a chronic medical condition such as diabetes.

Hydrate. Always drink plenty of water. Water is an essential nutrient involved in every function of the body. Water also helps maintain proper body temperature during a workout.

Don't overdo it. Extreme workouts are the trend in fitness, but be careful not to overdo it. The toll for over doing it is costly and becomes more costly as you age. Doing too much, too fast, too hard and too often leads us not to the question; "*If* you will get hurt," but rather "*When* you get hurt."

Find a partner. Enlisting the help of a friend on your fitness journey is a great tool. Having a friend to exercise with helps to keep you accountable and serves to motivate you. A workout partner not only makes the workout much more fun; buddies are great for giving encouragement and advice along your healthy lifestyle journey.

Warm up. A warm-up generally consists of a gradual increase in intensity in physical activity and joint mobility exercise, and stretching, followed by the exercise. No matter the exercise, a warm-up is needed. This helps to prevent strain and injuries.

Stretch. Stretching is good for both a warm-up and cool down. It increases flexibility and range of motion in the joints.

Tips For Maintaining Your Hair While Exercising:
Wrap it. Wrapping the hair around the head in a smooth form is called a "wrap." This is a good protective style for a workout. It helps to keep hair off of your face and neck. If your hair get slightly moist during a workout leave it wrapped

until the hair is dry. This will help the hair to maintain a smooth finish after the workout.

For shorter hair wrap a scarf around your hair. You don't have to cover your entire head, just wrap the scarf around your hairline, leaving the crown exposed. Ensure that the hair that is under the scarf is lying smooth before placing the scarf around the head. Failure to do so will cause the hair to set with the crinkle or disturbance. Tying the hair like this will preserve the volume without flattening your 'do.

Note: Although a cotton bandana helps to absorb perspiration, the bandanna also absorbs the natural moisture in your hair. If the head is completely covered in the bandana, the bandanna will trap in heat and cause more perspiration in the hair.

Style a Ponytail. Fashion a ponytail in the crown of your head. Don't allow the hair to rest on your neck. Doing so could be a distraction during your workout and may cause the hair to get wet from perspiration. Wearing an elastic band to match your outfit can be stylish and function to protect the hair from moisture.

Braid It. If your hair is long enough, braid it into one or two French braids, or simply one braided ponytail. You can then wrap it with a scarf or pin the braid or braids up. Post-workout, unravel the braids for a wavy look.

Wear a textured style. Curly styles or styles with texture are great options for working out. A wash n' go style is less time consuming than having to fully straighten hair after a workout. A bone straight style is likely to frizz during a workout but a textured look will endure a workout better.

Shampoo and condition often. A good workout that gets the heart rate up and blood circulating also causes perspiration. As we perspire we are eliminating toxins. These toxins along with sweat are drying to the hair and must be eliminated. Shampoo the hair on a frequent basis to rid hair of pollutants and to add moisture. It is a good idea to use a cleansing shampoo. If your hair is dry, alternate between moisturizing and cleansing shampoos. Always follow with a conditioner to replenish the moisture.

Avoid excessive heat. After a workout there is a temptation to "revive" your locks with heated tools, but do so with caution. Chemically treated hair is more prone to drying after a workout and heated tools can exacerbate the problem. Also, hair that is not clean is three times more likely to burn. If you use heated tools after a workout, turn down the heat!

Keeping the mane chic and attractive is always ideal, but the most attractive feature you have is a healthy and confident you. Working out can present challenges for your hair, but work through it. You are worth it!

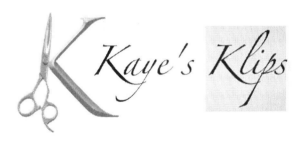

Because most toxins are stored in fat cells, when you start a new fat burning regimen, you may temporarily increase the amount of toxins in the blood stream. This often explains the tired, sluggish feeling when starting a new workout regimen.

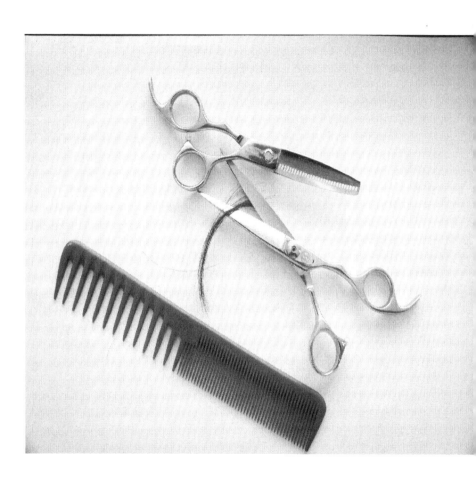

Chapter VI
Making the Cut!

Have you ever run into an old friend and heard the statement, "You look exactly the same" or "You haven't changed a bit?" My question is, was that a compliment?? Maybe. The statement could be translated that you are maintaining your youth – or it could have been an indication that you are stuck in a time machine. Everything must change . . . even your hairstyle.

Nothing dates you and screams boring like wearing the same hairstyle for years. Complacency is the greatest rival to change. We tend to find styles and trends that work well for us and are easy to maintain, and before you know it -- *voila'* -- years have passed. This saying may seem a bit dramatic, but it is true: Anything that doesn't change is soon obsolete or becomes an antique.

Earlier we established that your personal image says a lot to others about you. Failing to update your look suggests to others that you are not evolving and growing; instead, you are stagnant. Although other ways to refute that idea are at our disposal, a new hairstyle is an easy way to convey that you are a person of modern thought and fashion relevance.

For years a hairstyle meant lots of teasing, backcombing, curling and spraying. In the 60's and 70's Vidal Sassoon put more ease in hairstyling by designing cuts that were simple to maintain and became iconic styles. Today, most often a new style means a new haircut.

Is it time for a refresher? If not, great! If so, there is no better time than now. (See Appendix A to take a **Refresher Quiz** to determine if you need a hair refresher). Selecting a new, stylish haircut is strategic. You have to pick a style that will look nice and vogue on you, take a few years off your face and add polish; yet isn't labor intensive.

Selecting a new hairdo may seem scary and complicated, yet apps and websites are available that are designed to help you find the perfect haircut. If you are still unsure, here are a few tips to simplify the process:

Determine your style. What words best describes you? Fun and flirty? Simple and classic? Bold and adventurous? Smart and powerful? A great starting point is to know you; know your image or the image you would like to convey. This knowledge is important because *your* style might be simple and classic, but *your stylist* is thinking fun and whimsical.

Have a point of reference! Have an idea concerning how much hair you want to cut. Ask yourself how much time you want to devote to styling your hair. The best point of reference is a photo. If you are not exactly sure, have several pictures of cuts that you like. Be prepared to tell the stylist what you like most about the cut.

Consider you! Knowing your hair type, texture, density and face shape are important factors to consider when determining a haircut. Pick a style that works with your hair's texture. Hair comes in a variety of textures - from limp and silky thin hair to frizzy and bouncy coarse hair - and you should style yours accordingly. The right haircut should make you feel more confident and attractive. It should highlight your best features and downplay your flaws.

For example, a short and choppy cut that works on straight, thin hair won't look good on someone with thick and curly hair. Here are some general guidelines.

If you have fine, limp hair avoid wearing it in a long, blunt cut because that style can make you look child-like. Instead, favor volume-creating layers and try a shorter cut that hits at your shoulders or above. Never blunt cut bangs; opt instead for a side swept look.

If you have thick, coarse hair with a natural curl or wave, don't cut it too short - you'll end up with "Christmas tree" hair that's full and bushy at the bottom before tapering up to the head. Hair that's prone to frizz usually needs a little length to weigh it down. Consider cuts that start at the chin or below, and go longer if your hair is frizzier.

Find a compromise. For instance, if you've found a really great cut that you think would look flattering on your square face but you're worried about wearing thin hair long, ask your stylist if there's any way to add some volume. Your stylist will be happy to work with you and design the right look for you.

Know your face type and find a hairstyle that compliments your face. Weight, volume and length can really change the illusion of facial features. Generally, a good rule to follow is that you want your hair to be in opposition to the shape of your face. For example, on a really narrow face, add volume to make the face appear fuller; but on a square face, you should balance your sharp angles with soft layers or waves.

To determine your face shape, pull all your hair away from your face, take a photo of yourself and print it out on disposable paper. Next, trace the outline of your face. Compare your outline with the shapes below to determine your facial shape.

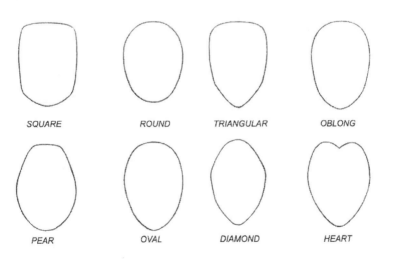

SQUARE   ROUND   TRIANGULAR   OBLONG

PEAR   OVAL   DIAMOND   HEART

Square faces are characterized by a broad forehead and wide cheekbones that square off at the jawbone. Blunt-cut bangs and cuts with sharp lines will make the jawline more pronounced.

Softer styles that balance the face are good choices for this shape. Consider long, sleek cuts and soft layers. Soft layers that frame the face are also a good balance for this facial shape. If you chose bangs, go with a side swept bang; bangs cut straight across will only box in your face.

Round faces are easily detected with the smoothly curved lines on both the hairline and chin. The forehead and chin are both a bit wide, with slightly wider cheekbones.

For this face shape, short hairstyles often give that "chubby cheek" look. Thus, round faces are best balanced by hairstyles that fall below the chin. The goal is to add length, keeping the hair close to the face which makes the face appear thinner. A hairstyle with height also helps with slimming out the face. A good idea is a long bob, or soft, adapted layers that are shoulder length.

Triangular faces are marked by a small forehead, with broader cheeks and chin. The triangular face is often referred to as pear-shaped. When choosing a style for this face shape, it's a good idea to find a style that will make the forehead appear broader. Soft bangs or a fringe will help to make the forehead appear fuller. Short haircuts with a lot of volume at the temples and in the top are ideal for triangular faces. You can also choose a longer cut, as long as it falls below the jawline.

Oblong faces maintain the same proportion throughout - the forehead, cheekbones and chin share about the same narrow width. The cheeks are usually sunken and the goal is to make the face appear fuller and shorter. Avoid long, straight styles and styles with a lot of height because those looks give the illusion that the face is even longer. Bobs and styles with fullness will make the face appear fuller. Curls and waves work well in adding width.

Oval faces are considered the ideal face shape. In comparison to the round face shape it is similar in proportion to round, but more elongated with a little less width in the checks. The forehead is slightly wider than the chin, with distinct lines from the cheekbones going down to the chin. Most hairstyles work for this face structure. In this case, find the feature you want to highlight with your hairstyle. For example if you want to highlight your eyes, bangs will draw attention to them.

Note: *If you have a great bone structure you can wear almost any style, but a short cut makes a bold statement. However, if your neck is short, try to keep your hair long because short hair draws attention to your neckline.*

Diamond-shaped faces are defined by a narrow chin and forehead, with broad cheeks. Try to create width at the forehead with bangs, and reduce the width across the cheeks with layers that start at the chin. Avoid hairstyles that move away from the face or that rest behind the ear.

Heart-shaped faces are the opposite of triangular faces. This facial shape is defined primarily by a wide forehead and narrow or pointy chin. The cheekbones may be about the same width as the forehead or slightly wider. The goal is to decrease the width of the forehead, thus bangs work well at balancing out this facial shape. Side swept bangs or bangs snipped straight across the forehead work well. A short cut is also a good choice. Keep the hair close to the head with little to no volume and avoid choppy layers that hit at the chin.

Note: If you are still unsure about a look that fits your facial shape, look at some of the hairstyles of others with your same facial shape.

Additional tips to consider when selecting a new hair cut:

Be verbal. It is important to your stylist that you love your new look, yet your stylist cannot read your mind. If you have questions, thoughts or concerns, **speak up**. Communication is very essential in accomplishing your new look. If the style is not exactly what you want, just say so! It's very possible that what you want will come as an easy fix for your stylist.

Listen to the expert. Although you should have an idea of what you want, sometimes the professional will have suggestions or ideas that you haven't considered. Stylists are also experienced at knowing what works best for your hair type and texture. Ask your stylist if he/she thinks the style will work for you. If the stylist disagrees with the hairstyle you have in mind, simply ask the stylist to explain why. Remember, your stylist is a trained professional – please value and respect his/her opinion!

Consider the maintenance. How much time every day are you willing to spend styling your new 'do? Will you have to blow-dry or use a flat iron? Layers require more maintenance than a blunt cut. Short hairstyles will need to be cut often to maintain the length, but with longer hair special attention must be given to avoiding heat damage and split ends. Will your new hairstyle work with your lifestyle? Considering maintenance is paramount because no matter how great the cut is, if it's too high maintenance you will soon become weary of that hairstyle.

Accent with color. The perfect complement to any haircut is color. Coloring your hair can be high-maintenance, but the right color that is strategically placed will serve as a great feature. Selecting the right shade and tone can be tricky, so consult your stylist about which color would look best on you. In the next chapter we will present a more in-depth discussion of color.

Count to 10! Never decide to get a drastic cut when you are angry or upset. Often you will come to regret your rash decision – and waiting for the hair to grow back can be quite frustrating!

Note: If you are not sure about cutting your hair, start small. You can always cut more, but when you cut too much, you just have to wait for your hair to grow back.

Find a good hairstylist. Once you know you have a stylist you can trust with your hair, getting a haircut becomes a lot less stressful. Do some research and find a quality professional that is willing to listen to your ideas and accurately assess your needs. It might cost a little more up-front, but you'll save money in the long run when you don't have to go to someone else to fix a bad haircut.

These considerations should guide you to the perfect cut, but life has no guarantees. Sometimes bad haircuts happen to good people! What happens if you go in a salon, ask for a specific look and you leave looking like your hair was cut with a lawn mower?? I know your first thought is to scream and cry profusely like your life is over.

After you get past the initial shock, here are a few tips for **getting past a bad haircut:**

Get your hair evenly cut. Visit another salon to have it cut evenly, because if your hair starts out uneven, it grows back uneven. Cut it some more so it will be a nice look as it grows out. If it is too short to cut, now wait until it grows out more and then have it cut even.

Accessorize. Wearing beautiful and ornate hair accessories will deflect attention from your cut.

Experiment! Try new products or curling it differently; doing this may help you to enjoy your hair better.

Add color. A fabulous new color can add new dimension and life to a bad haircut.

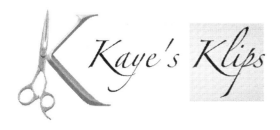

Finding a stylist that you can trust and that communicates well with you is the first step to a great cut.

Here are a few tips to bridging the communication gap with your stylist:

1. Find a qualified stylist who understands hair care **and** customer service. If the stylist is not given to providing good customer service then it will be difficult to make him/her **hear** you.

2. If you are visiting a new stylist, ask her/him concerning their areas of expertise. Most stylists have a specialty. Some stylists are great at color but not so good at cutting, and vice versus. Your desired look may not be their forte. It's best to visit a stylist who produces the type of look you desire.

3. During the consultation; **be firm but CLEAR about what you want.** Let photos be your PRIMARY mouthpiece. Because they are non-

professionals, clients often will use the wrong terminology and thus misguide the stylist. Let any verbal instructions be precise and as descriptive as possible. It is also a good idea to say what you **DON'T** want.

4. Ask your stylist what he/she suggests. Communication is a two-way street. Respect your stylist's opinions and expertise; this makes it easier for them to respect yours.

5. Listen carefully to the stylist. If he/she suggests something that concerns you, don't be shy about asking more questions. If the stylist seems to be overlooking some of your concerns, restate your questions and ask him/her to address your concern.

6. After you have settled on a style, have the stylist to repeat the plan of action so you can be sure that the two of you are in agreement!

Choosing a stylist that values you as a client and is interested in your needs is very important. Every stylist wants you to be happy; often all they need is to hear from you is to know exactly what you want. Don't assume that your stylist understands what you want, **yet don't be insulting** when you communicate what you want. It's never a good idea to offend a stylist before they work on your hair. If you are willing to make the commitment to developing good communication with your stylist, the rewards will definitely be worth it!

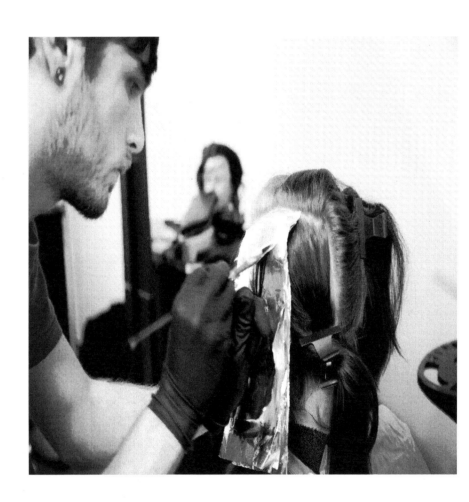

Chapter VII
Dyeing to Color

Do you want something new? Are you bursting at the seams, dying to get some color? Maybe you want to totally reinvent yourself or just add a little flavor. Either way, coloring your hair is guaranteed to change your look. In most cases color seems to take a few years off of your look.

Forty was once said to be the new 30; now 50 appears to be the new 30. It seems that we are getting younger and younger. We are constantly in search of the fountain of youth. Do you remember a time when all adults seemed archaic? Why has that changed? Some of it has to do with the fact that as you age, your perception of age changes. These days, most of us are living better and taking better care of ourselves. One of the biggest changes in how we take care of ourselves involves hair color.

One report indicated that 30 years ago, only 20% of the adult population wore hair color; **today almost 70% of the adult population wears color**.

Let's face it; wearing grey hair makes most people look older, and mousy blonde is just boring. The questions have been asked, "Do blondes really have more fun? Are brunettes more sage? Or, do redheads have more spice?" I'm not sure there is a definitive answer to those questions, and we won't seek to explore them now. What *is* clear is that "colored" (hair) girls tend to look more youthful and polished.

The truth is, girls are not the only ones wearing haircolor. In fact, an increasing number of men have taken to coloring their hair. Haircolor can be that amazing magic wand that instantly transforms a Plane Jane into the Belle of the Ball or transpose the frog into the handsome prince. Haircolor does so much more than cover grey. It is used to add dimension to hair and make fine, limp hair look fuller. Haircolor is a form of self-expression and is often used to highlight a particular haircut or facial feature.

Although haircolor has transformative power, it should not be taken lightly; it is a chemical service. Coloring the hair is much more complex than it appears, because several factors must be taken into consideration when formulating color. A color service combines the deepest artistic expressions of a stylist, the workmanship of a masterful surgeon and the precision of science. For many coloring the hair is very

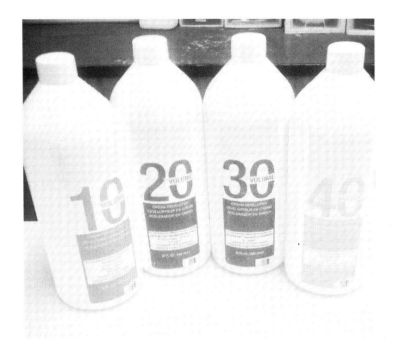

confusing and to gain a full understanding requires some patience. For this reason, I personally recommend that hair coloring be reserved for a professional colorist.

However; for those adventurous DIY hair enthusiasts or for those wanting to experiment on the most basic level, let me take some of the mystery out of color:

What is Hair Color?

Hair Color is a solution that is used to dye, tint or lighten one's hair.

*Note: Hair color refers to a person's natural color of hair. The term **Haircolor** refers to artificial hair color products and services.*

Five Types Of Haircolor:

Natural / Vegetable Dyes

Natural or vegetable dyes are colorants derived from plants, berries, insects and minerals. Most natural dyes are vegetable dyes which are obtained from plant sources –roots, berries, bark, leaves, wood — and other organic sources. The use of natural dyes dates as far back as 3000 B.C. when ancient Egyptians used henna colors to stain their hair and nails.

 Henna's or natural dyes or extremely safe to use on hair, but there are a few drawbacks:

-They do not lighten hair, they only stain hair.

-The colors available are very limited.

-The process is lengthy with little impact.

-Most chemical color services can't be applied over natural colors.

Temporary Color

Temporary color does not penetrate the hair shaft; instead, it coats the hair. As suggested by the name, temporary color is temporary and usually lasts until the next shampoo. A temporary color comes in the form of a spray, foam or mousse, shampoo, gel or mascara.

Semi-Permanent Color

Semi-permanent color is designed to last longer than a temporary color. This type of color lasts four to six weeks depending on the porosity of the hair and how often you shampoo. Semi-permanent color doesn't have ammonia, and does not require any mixing. These colors cannot *lighten* hair, they only deposit color or "stain" the hair. Because semi-permanent color rinses out with each shampoo, it is best to first shampoo the hair, towel dry and then apply the semi-permanent color or rinse.

Demi-permanent color

Demi-permanent color is a deposit only color. They usually have a much lower pH than colors that lighten. Demi-permanent colors are mixed with a developer, but a low volume developer. This is designed to raise the cuticle slightly so the color can be deposited. Demi-permanent color does not lighten hair, which makes it an excellent choice for covering the grey.

Permanent Color

Permanent color is a highly alkaline product designed to permanently change natural hair color. The color contains an ammonia. When mixed with developer (in various volumes, 10, 20, 30, and 40; note that 30 and 40 volumes are reserved for professional use only), it opens the cuticle layer of hair. This allows the peroxide to actually lighten hair while the color deposits color molecules into the hair. Permanent haircolor is used to lighten natural color, change color or cover grey.

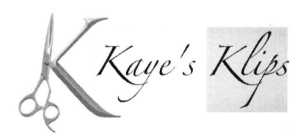

Though bleaching your hair is common - do not try this at home! Never under estimate the process. Bleach is not a haircolor, it is actually a

*"decolorizer," meaning you remove **all** pigment from hair. The process of bleaching compromises the integrity of the hair, and must be maintained with the gentlest of treatments.*

When buying color there are a few things you should know.

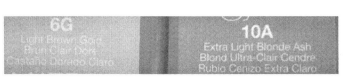

Most colors refer to both a number and letter; for example, 6G/ Dark Golden Brown or 10A/ Light Ash Blonde. The *number* refers to the level of lightness and the *letter* refers to the tone. You should understand both before considering coloring hair.

LEVEL

Level refers to the degree of lightness or darkness of a color. Each color family has light, medium and dark levels; for example, light brown, medium brown and dark brown. While each haircolor brand has its own system of identifying levels and tones, the natural hair color levels range form 1-10.

This chart should serve as a starting point to help you identify hair color levels:

10. Lightest blonde

9. Light Blonde

8. Blonde

7. Medium Blonde

6. Dark blonde

5. Light Brown

4. Medium Brown

3. Dark Brown

2. Off Black

1. Black

TONE

Tone refers to the hue or shade of hair. It also refers to its degree of warmth or coolness. Tones are categorized as warm, neutral or cool, and are usually part of the shade description (think terms like "gold" or "ash"). No matter what your level of color, you can choose from a variety of tones to help you achieve your color transformation.

Refer to this chart for a description of some common tones:

A / ASH (Cool) - Color which uses green/blue color pigments.

N / NEUTRAL - Color which has an equal amount of primary color pigments (balanced).

C / COPPER - (Warm) - Color which adds reds and yellow pigments to create orange.

B /BEIGE - Similar to a neutral, but may be warmer or cool, depending on base.

G / GOLD (Warm) - Color which adds gold pigments.

R / RED (Warm) - Color which adds red pigments.

M / MOCHA (Warm) - Brown color with warm pigments.

Before you color:

- Ensure that there are no existing abrasions on your scalp. Don't brush or aggravate your scalp before applying permanent hair color.

- Start with healthy hair. If your hair is already fragile, applying permanent hair color will further compromise the integrity of your hair.

- Apply a thin layer of Vaseline or some protective cream around the hairline to protect the skin from staining.
- If your skin is stained by the color, don't panic! Most beauty supply stores sell hair color stain removers; these work well to cleanse the skin of any residual color.
- Be careful to cover your hair strands fully to ensure even color penetration.
- Semi-permanent colors, demi-permanent colors and vegetable dyes will not lighten hair; they will only deposit color, cover grey, or change the hue of your hair. These are always the safest to use.
- Don't get too creative and stray away from the directions on the box. Pay close attention to the recommended timing.

Educator and Creative Artistic Team Member for global Farouk®, Incorporated for several years, Sami G offers the following color tips to help you with some of your color challenges:

♥Most manufacturers' color lines are a shade darker than salon quality products. If you know your level from a salon standpoint then use a level darker when purchasing a store product.

♥Tone also makes a huge difference. Remember that all of your "N" colors are best for covering grey. They contain all three primary colors so they will grab your grey hair better. You can add a tone to your formula to enhance color. For example, if you use a level 8 Gold in a salon, then at the store look for a level 9NG if you have grey and want to accent the gold.

♥Most box colors come with a 20-volume peroxide to process the color. IF you want to darken hair or just deepen your color (called a demi-permanent, or deposit-only color), chose a level lighter than yours. Then empty half of the bottle of 20-volume peroxide/developer and add water to it. Water dilutes the 20-volume developer into a 10-volume developer which is used to deposit color only.

♥Reds are the hardest color to keep and maintain. The red molecule is the largest of the colors and does not replace the color molecule in the natural hair. It only stains the hair and slightly deposits color into the hair shaft, therefore it will not need to be refreshed often.

♥To help maintain color, especially reds, use a glaze to boost vibrancy and shine.

♥Root touch-up kits are very reliable to use. Since you are only coloring your roots it's very easy to match your natural color. Generally with a touch-up kit you are able to use the same level you use at a salon or a shade darker. Grey hair tends to look a shade lighter anyway so a darker shade would suffice.

♥If you color your hair too dark - don't stress! You can purchase a stripping kit at the grocery store. Use as directed. You may have to strip your hair up to four times to remove all of the color. **YOU CANNOT** color your hair the same day you strip. Molecules of the old color are still present although it looks lighter. These molecules will react to new dye and take it back to the color you stripped. **You have to wait four-five days for the hair to oxidize, before you are able to color you hair again.**

♥Highlighting kits are great for lighter colors of hair. Level 6 or higher, which is a lightest brown, will highlight beautifully with at home kits. If you are darker than a level 6 then DO NOT use these kits because you will produce orangey color highlights on darker levels. These levels must seek a professional to highlight successfully.

♥Never use a color with an ash or violet tone/base on blonde hair when wanting to go darker. These colors produce a mossy color on blonde hair. You must use a gold-based color to darken blonde hair. Remember to dilute the peroxide with water before mixing and coloring.

♥Color correction should be best left to the hands of a professional, but IF you ever want to fix a color you must refer to the color wheel. Opposite colors will neutralize each other and help you to remove unwanted tones. So, if your hair is green then you should use a color with red in it. Red is opposite of green on a color wheel and will neutralize or balance the color.

♥If your hair has previously been chemically treated with a permanent wave or a chemical relaxer, then **DO NOT** attempt an at home color. Chemically treated hair is more fragile because it has already been compromised; adding color is a delicate procedure and should be saved for a color specialist.

After you have achieved a beautiful color, Sami G offers these maintenance tips to keeps your locks full of luster:

♥Always use a shampoo that is labeled sulfate free or low sulfates. Sulfates have a stripping action and can strip your color at a faster rate.

♥Always rinse your conditioner in cold water. Cold water allows the hair to close and capture conditioner in the hair, thus making it stronger.

♥Avoid exposing your hair to the sun. The sun is a natural hair lightener, and overexposure can cause hair to fade or even change colors.

♥Olive oil is nature's miracle conditioner. Apply olive oil to dry hair and sleep with a shower cap and it conditions extremely dry hair. Shampoo the oil out the next day.

♥To keep your color longer; use a leave-in conditioning spray treatment. This treatment has a lower pH and will tighten the cuticle to keep your hair color longer. Shampoo and condition your hair as usual, then lightly spray in the leave-in conditioner and style as usual.

Color presents limitless possibilities. These tips should serve as a starting point to help open that world of potentiality. Whether you're "dyeing" to color in a bolder, more adventurous hue or dyeing to cover roots; color adds richness, shine and excitement but should never be taken lightly. ~SG

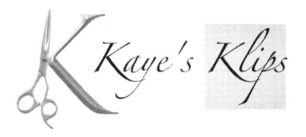

Professional Consultants and Resources for the Beauty and Salon Industry (PCR) reported $756,000,000 was spent in the United States on the purchase of haircolor in 2012. Haircolor is booming business and growing in popularity. It appears we are all "dyeing to color!"

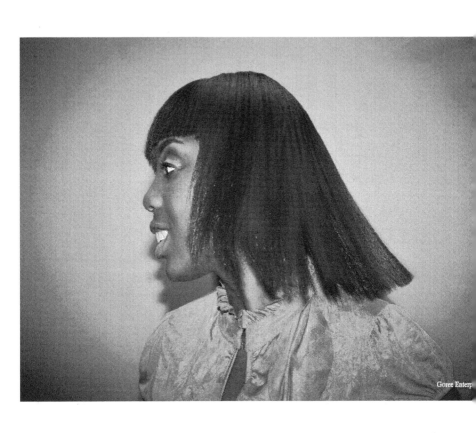

Chapter VIII
Relax: Natural or Straight

A chemical relaxer, often referred to as a perm, is a service that is designed to chemically rearrange or "relax" extremely curly hair to a straighter and smoother form.

Relaxers date back to the early 1900's, when Garret Morgan realized that lye could relax curls. However, because the lye was very uncomfortable to the skin and extremely damaging to the hair, relaxers didn't have commercial appeal. Although there were small improvements to the formulations, relaxers were primarily home concoctions that used a mix of lye and soap.

Hair relaxers changed in the 1970's. The Pro-Line® Corporation introduced the first commercially produced lye relaxer. Soon, the Johnson Products® Company introduced the first no-lye relaxer – and it was a "game-changer." Johnson Products® was able to gain footage in the industry because they were the first company to sponsor a television show geared to Black entertainment. Every week when African Americans turned on the *Soul Train* show, they saw commercials for Gentle Treatment No-Lye Relaxer® and reminded of how we could have "bouncing and behaving hair." This commercial saturation revolutionized the Black hair care industry.

I watched as the relaxer gained momentum. I remember a time when 100% of my Mom's clients were "natural." They either got a press or wore an Afro. As I think back on my early childhood; it triggers images of walking in her salon seeing it full of smoke. No, not cigarette smoke; instead, this was smoke permeated from all of the burning grease in the pressed hair. Eventually, my Mom's clientele transitioned from 100% natural to approximately 85% of her clients wearing a relaxer upon her retirement.

The 80's and 90's were great times for manufacturing companies that produced relaxers. The popularity of the relaxer was phenomenal. But soon after the turn of the century, Black women started to consider the idea of abandoning the relaxer and embracing their natural curls. Again, this was another trend in hair care that I have had the pleasure of watching unfold.

At the onset of the natural hair movement, women who were bold enough to embrace their natural curls were seen as defiant, militant and even in some settings, unkempt. Hair care manufacturers totally ignored requests for products that catered to natural hair. Refusing to be denied, a few entrepreneurs took to their kitchens and began to experiment with products.

The Internet became an outlet to discuss natural hair care needs and products; and the movement began to grow. In 2007 Chris Rock produced a movie, *Good Hair* where he explored a manufacturing plant that produces sodium hydroxide, which is an ingredient used in most relaxers. In the movie, Chris Rock showed a Coke® can being dissolved in sodium hydroxide. This was a powerful image, and even more women began to move away from relaxers.

In response to the image of sodium hydroxide I will say, although it was powerful, I believe it was an unfair representation. Sodium hydroxide in its purest form is indeed a strong alkali product, but it's rarely used in full concentration. The highest concentration of sodium hydroxide used in any relaxer formulation was 10%. Today, most relaxer systems contain as little as 2-5% of sodium hydroxide in their formulations, with the rest of the formula containing buffers, emollients and conditioners.

Sodium hydroxide is recognized by most as the principal strong alkali (base) in chemistry. It is used in most cases where the desired result is to neutralize an acid or raise the alkalinity of a product. Though it can be extremely harmful, when balanced, it losses it intensity. Did you know that sodium hydroxide is a key ingredient in the purification process of drinking water? I don't say this to discount the dangers associated with chemical relaxers, rather I say this to point out that when used in proper balance, sodium hydroxide can be safe enough to drink.

I understand the concerns for relaxer safety, and I have them too. Routinely I speak with clients that are disgruntled with relaxers. Upon closer review, I see where they repeatedly made several costly mistakes that are hazardous to hair health. Instead of acknowledging their mistakes, they conclude that relaxers alone were the culprit. There are dangers associated with hair relaxers and as consumers; you should not underestimate those dangers. It is important that you follow all safety and hair health precautions.

I am often asked about my preference for natural or relaxed hair, the sustainability of the relaxer, the dangers of sodium hydroxide and the future of the Black hair care industry. Concerning my preference, I will start by saying, as a hairstylist I love hair! I like hair long, medium, or short. I like textured hair and curly hair; I also like it straight. Hair can be red, brunette, blonde, or somewhere in between. I like a dazzling, ornate up-do as much as a clean side-swept ponytail. From the artistic and visually stimulating value of cornrows, to the awe-inspiring afro or a classic bob; the list goes on and on. I do not discriminate, I love hair! I see the beauty in **all** hair.

When talking about the future of the Black hair care industry, I know that nothing stays the same and hair care as we know it today is destined to change. However, I know that hair artistry is an ancient practice that will remain. How it will evolve, I am not sure, but I will be here making an impact and enjoying it all!

So now let's take a look at relaxers and natural hair. Many women of color face the choice: Straighten or remain natural. It's not an easy, cut-and-dried decision. They both have their unique benefits and require a considerable amount of maintenance. I will not seek to persuade you on either; I will simply present the facts as I know them. By presenting the facts and telling you the pros and cons, I hope to help you make your own choice based on good information.

Chemical Relaxers

A relaxer is a product designed chemically to relax the natural curl in highly textured hair; leaving the hair softer, smoother, less tangled and straighter. The active ingredient in traditional relaxers is Sodium Hydroxide (lye) which raises the cuticle, allowing the product to penetrate the cortex and straighten the hair. Once the procedure is complete the hair is rinsed and shampooed with a neutralizing (acid balancing) shampoo and a conditioner is applied to replenish the natural moisture lost during the relaxing process. Following the recommended timing guide for your hair texture is very important.

As new hair grows in, it is un-relaxed. To maintain the relaxer, the new growth is retouched as needed. During the retouch, the relaxer is applied to new growth only. Overlapping previously relaxed hair severely comprises the integrity of the hair and can cause breakage. The average retouch application is every six-to-eight weeks.

Because relaxing is a chemical service, it is highly recommended that this service be performed by a professional stylist only. There is always a risk of danger when using any type of chemicals, so careful attention in the application process is crucial. Professional stylists are even encouraged to have the service performed by another professional to avoid overlapping and minimize risks.

Base and No-Base Formulas

The terms "base" and "no base" refer to the need to apply a light protective covering (usually petroleum jelly) on the scalp to minimize irritation. No-base relaxers have reduced concentrations of sodium hydroxide (lye) and can come in contact with the skin and scalp without much irritation. Although more and more relaxers are "no base," most manufactures realize there is still some potential risk of irritation. Thus, using a base cream is encouraged as a preventative measure.

No-Lye Relaxer

When relaxers began to enjoy commercial sales, sodium hydroxide, also known as lye was the active ingredient. Because of the irritation and harshness associated with traditional relaxers, alternative straightening ingredients were created. Potassium hydroxide, calcium hydroxide, guanidine hydroxide and lithium hydroxide are slightly weaker alkaline agents than sodium hydroxide, yet they produce very similar results in relaxing. Although gentler on the scalp, they tend to strip the hair more of natural oils and require a larger number of moisturizing conditioners to balance the hair.

These alternate hydroxide relaxers are not as stable as sodium hydroxide. As a result they are not sold pre-mixed; instead they require being mixed at the time of use. The formula is most reliable when it is first mixed; after mixing, the relaxer has a shelf life of 24 to 48 hours. (Check the manufacturer's recommendations). Calcium and guanidine hydroxide are commonly used in sensitive scalp formulas because they are gentler to the skin.

Benefits And Risks Of Relaxer

♥Most relaxers have conditioners and moisturizers built in the system. As a result, the hair is not only straightened, it retains moisture better.

♥The relaxer offers flexibility in styling options. Though relaxed hair can still be styled to mimic a natural curl, relaxers offer ease in maintaining a variety of sleek and straight styles.

♥By straightening the natural curl, the relaxer assists in managing frizz and tangles.

♥The biggest risk is breakage or hair loss. With any chemical, there is always a risk of damage of over processing.

♥The cost of salon visits and in-home maintenance can cause a strain on your budget.

♥Scalp irritation (which can be very uncomfortable) is a common side effect of relaxing the hair.

♥The overall maintenance for a relaxer is more detailed. It requires routine reconstructive and moisturizing conditioners.

♥When the hair is relaxed, extreme caution is advised when attempting another chemical service such as color, because the integrity of the hair has already been compromised with the relaxer.

By observing the following safety tips, you will experience better results and a healthier mane outcome:

♥Check the scalp to ensure that there are no prior abrasions, cuts, scrapes, bruises or irritations.

♥Apply a protective cream to protect the scalp and on the hair to shield it against overlapping.

♥Ensure not to overlap product on previously relaxed hair.

♥Refrain from relaxing hair that has been previously lightened with bleach.

♥Select the formula and strength that best fits your hair texture.

♥Follow the recommended processing time. **It is not a good idea to wait until the relaxer starts to "burn;" instead, stick closely to the recommended processing time.**

♥Rinse thoroughly to remove chemicals from the hair. If the products are not totally removed from the hair, there is no automatic shut-off; it continues processing, causing extreme damage to the hair.

♥Always use neutralizing shampoo after each application to close the cuticle and balance the pH.

♥Don't get creative in the use of relaxers or the rules of application. It is important to follow the manufacturer's instructions.

Natural Hair
~by Deshonica Kerrie, Design Essentials® Educator and Natural Hair Specialist

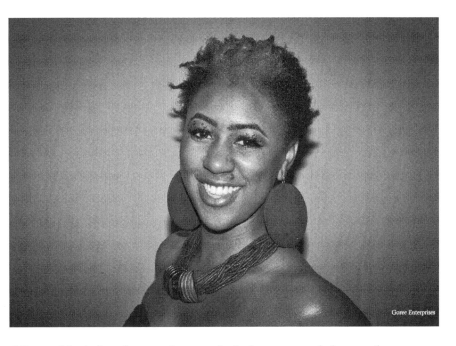

Goree Enterprises

Natural hair has been a hot topic in homes and the work place, with friends and in schools. It is an old topic with a new feel, and lifelong naturalists stand in awe of the new boom of the natural presence in the world. Some think it's a trend and some think it's a movement, yet those that have embarked upon the natural hair journey realize it's a way of life. This is not the beginning or the end, natural hair has been here and is here to stay!

So What Exactly Is Natural Hair?

There are a few definitions for natural hair. **Some define it as your unaltered, God-given hair as it grows through the epidermis from follicles deep within the dermis.** The hair is not chemically altered, colored, curled or straightened by relaxers, texturizers or other chemical agents and is free of any and all extensions. Colored hair is sometimes considered natural, yet this definition depends on who does the defining. It is important to note that repeated hair coloring *does* alter the texture slightly; this is why some believe that hair with haircolor is not completely "natural."

Another interesting definition for natural hair is **virgin hair** - Hair whose texture hasn't been altered by chemical straighteners, including relaxers and texturizers.

Any hair type or texture that hasn't been chemically processed is virgin, but the term "natural" hair usually refers to African American or Black hair.

An Afro is sometimes referred to as a "natural," but natural hair can be adorned in many other styles besides a "fro." Pressed hair is still considered natural because once shampooed, the texture returns to its unaltered state.

As a natural hair care specialist, I have personally concluded that to be "natural" is to embrace the texture you were born with. Being "natural" means you understand that we are all born with different textures. The ability to embrace your texture it is a valuable lesson, because in some cases one head of hair may be composed of different textures.

Natural hair care is not new, nor is the choice for everyone, but when I transition a client to natural, it is because we have determined it to be a better choice for that client.

Consider these points when transitioning to natural:

Be open. If you have not transitioned to natural, have an open mind.

Carefully consider your choice so that you make an informed decision; one the fits your lifestyle.

Patience is imperative! The process is time consuming and requires diligence.

Practicing in the industry since 1992, I have studied the pros and cons of both chemically treated and natural hair. I have realized that too much of one thing and not enough of something else can *each* pose a negative effect. Having an open mind, conducting research of both chemically treated and natural hair, and studying proper application of natural hair products and techniques – or chemicals – can help ensure you have more pros then cons when making the choice that fits your lifestyle.

As a cosmetologist that has embraced natural hair care, I have realized that stylists and people in the natural community speak different languages. This communication barrier has driven a wedge between the two communities. The natural community has taken to doing their hair at home and prefer to "do-it-yourself; also known as DIY. This DIY mindset came about as a result of stylists' overuse of chemicals and their neglect to give attention to natural hair care needs. Some poor stylist have shown such a blatant disregard for naturalists and their hair journey that this attitude has shattered naturals' trust in stylists.

On the other hand, some stylists are offended and feel minimized because of the misconceptions and misunderstandings of natural hair and how to care for it. It is important to note that cosmetology is the emergence of art, science, and innate talent, and stylists believe that reading things doesn't make a naturalist an expert. Besides, everything you read on the Internet is not true!

Some naturalists may also opt to use relaxers and texturizers that are designed to give more control yet not completely straighten the hair. If you use these products in this way, take note that the processing time should not exceed manufactures instructions. Additionally, depending on the hair that you are working with, the processing time may also be considerably less than is stated on the package.

I really enjoy natural hair and seeing more people, both men and women being more comfortable with wearing their natural hair and embracing it. The key is patience; it is one of the main ingredients to understanding what your hair can do.

Eating well, working out, laughing, not stressing and being positive are all great ways to continue to grow your natural hair.

Understanding the type and texture of your natural hair will also help you understand product selection. Yes, I know.... there are so many products to choose from and it's a challenge not to become a product junkie!

This is where trial and error will come in. This is also a time to connect with a professional cosmetologist to help you understand the needs of your hair. Of course, no one understands your hair better then you; however, as cosmetologists we can assist you with the knowledge we possess that may be beyond your reach.

This chart may give a clear understanding of the curl reference chart so the cosmetologist as well as the DIY-ers may be on the same page. The hair characteristics listed in this chart should also assist you in the product selection as well as some styling options:

Cosmetologist	DIYers	Hair Characteristics
Loose Wavy	2b	Very loose S wave form, limited body or volume prone to frizz
Wavy with curls	2c	Consistent S Wave with ringlet curls, moderate body or volume, frizz easily and resistant to styling
Curly with loops	3a	Distinct well defined S formed loops, lots of body and movement with good elasticity, excellent style and versatility
Curly with spirals	3b	Well defined curls of spiral ringlets with a natural spring, lots of body and may tangle, easy to swell, dry out and frizz
Curly with coils	3c	Well defined tight curls in corkscrew or coil shapes, highly dense and full of volume, easy to swell, tangle, and frizz and requires moisture
Coiled with spring	4a	Coiled with an evident S or ringlet pattern, some volume due to density but limited to movement
Tightly coiled	4b	Hair is extra tangled and requires extra moisture, tightly coiled with less defined curls, hair is highly dense and wiry, lacks movement, hair is fragile and requires moisture
Tightly Coiled with Zig Zag	4c	Very tightly coiled in a zigzag pattern, requires manipulation to achieve curl definition, hair is fragile and requires moisture, hair is dense and shrinks.

Here are some great benefits of having natural hair:

♥Embracing your natural curls makes your hair appear fuller.

♥You have the versatility of wearing your hair straight or curly.

♥By eliminating the chemical relaxer, you open your options to explore color more freely without the fear of double processing your hair.

♥Being natural enhances your ability to embrace the natural you! Loving the way your hair looks in its natural state, and understanding how to maintain it fosters more self-love.

Some of the concerns of going natural are:

♥Reluctance to go natural because you feel you have to fit into what society has classified as "beauty."

♥The time involved in styling and maintenance.

♥There are a vast number of natural products on the market. Finding the one that works best for your hair type can be challenging and costly.

♥The patience and dedication needed for the transitional phase is not easily obtained.

♥Proper hair shaping, conditioning, and proper use of color is very essential to having healthy natural hair.

In closing, I would like to state that my vision for the natural hair community as well as cosmetologists is that we work *together* to speak a language that we all understand: The **healthy hair** language. The reason this is so important is because we need each other and we can really learn from one another.

As I stated previously, life is about choices. Loving yourself from the inside out is very important for healthy living. Embracing every choice you make, even the ones you may not be able to control. Don't judge others for the simple choice of whether they relax their hair or not. Be you and do you, and don't let **anyone** make you feel uncomfortable with who you are. Stay positive and confident every day! ♥~DK

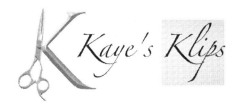

Mintel Oxygen, a marketing research firm, estimated the Black hair care market reached $684 million in 2012. In 2010, they estimated that 26% of African American Women had abandoned relaxers and were wearing their hair natural. In 2011 that percentage jumped by 10%, which is a noticeable increase. Mintel anticipates relaxer sales to plummet by 67% between 2011 and 2016.[11]

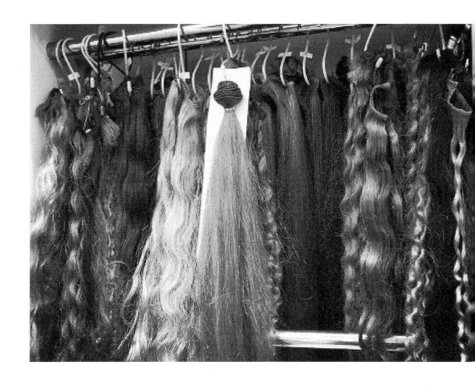

Chapter IX
Sew It or Grow It: Extensions 101
~By Ana Thomas, Owner of Good Hair & Co.

Many women dream of having longer and more voluminous hair. For some women, their "gene pool" will not let them realize that dream; for others, there is excitement at the idea of totally changing their look.

When your hair does not grow as fast or as thick as you would like, or if you want to add some spice or excitement to your look, hair extensions are an option. Available is a variety of lengths, textures, and colors; extensions allow every woman the opportunity to experience a level of versatility that her own hair may not offer her. **Hair extensions are methods of adding length or fullness to one's hair by adding commercial hair or weave.**

Extensions also serve as a protective hairstyle for women seeking alternatives to exposing their own hair to the extremes of heated tools or various climates. With the installation of extensions, the styling options are endless. The history of hairpieces traces back to the time of the ancient Egyptians, who used wigs when they would shave their heads to be more comfortable in the hot climate and decrease lice infestation. In the 17th century wigs dominated popular culture and fashion.

For centuries, hairpieces were exclusive to wealthy individuals. Since then much has changed. Extensions have secured a popular place in mainstream society. Many celebrities don expensive hairpieces that have caused women of all ethnicities to follow suit. Methods of applications, as well as types of hair have evolved tremendously. In most cases, a complete install can be performed in one visit with no discomfort to the client.

When choosing hair extensions, the color and texture of the hair are crucial considerations. The goal of hair extensions should be to produce a natural-looking result. In other words, no one should be able to tell your hair has extensions, unless you desire otherwise. The individual should choose hair extensions that match his or her own hair color and texture, such as straight and fine or curly and coarse.

Methods of Installation

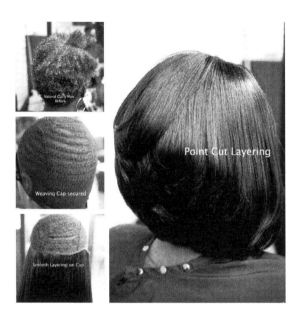

Braided Install: The most popular method of extension installation is the braided install, also known as the "sew in." The natural hair is braided in a pattern and the weave hair is sewn to the braids. The braiding pattern is the most important aspect of the install, because it will determine how the extensions will lay. They should lie flat, and fall in a natural hair flow.

A small portion of natural hair is left out in the crown area and around the perimeter to cover the extensions. This method is ideal if you are seeking to add length, volume, or experiment with a completely different texture. Braided installs can be worn eight to10 weeks with ease. Because there is no glue or adhesive involved, women are able to swim, work out or wash their hair without interrupting the install. This technique offers the most versatility.

Braidless Install: Braidless installs are ideal for women with fine or thinning hair. This method is the most natural extension service, as wefts lay very flat and natural when installed.

The average lifespan for the braidless install is six to eight weeks. This method is very similar to the braided sew in, but the foundations isn't composed of braids. Instead, small links, or micro links, are attached to the hair spaced apart in 1' increments. Wefts are then sewn to links in a single row. Micro-linking also doesn't involve any glue or adhesives; however, this method does require a bit more caution than the braided install due to the fragile nature of the installed links. If neglected, hair can become tangled in the micro links and cause breakage.

Bonded: Bonded extensions are one of the more temporary installations. Bonded to the scalp with a mild adhesive, wefts stay in place until the hair is shampooed. If seeking to add a quick hint of color, or volume in a specific area bonded wefts are a great choice. Proper removal is the most important aspect of this method. Removing adhered wefts without a proper removal cream could lead to extensive damage.

Clip-ins: This technique is the most temporary of the installations and can be applied with much ease. The hair weft has small hair clips sewn onto them. When applying clip-ins, the hair is sectioned neatly, and then the weft with the clips is placed onto this clean parting with the clips facing the scalp. Each clip is snapped into place. It can be helpful to backcomb lightly each section for a more secure grip. This process is repeated until each clip-in weft is in place.

To show the versatility of this type of hair extension, some choose to install clip-ins just for nightlife, while others wear them daily. Because of their temporary nature, clip-ins should be removed before bedtime and not be worn while asleep.

Tension is also another important factor in extension installation. A slight amount of tension is needed to secure the extensions. However, foundations for braided installs that are too tight or high in tension, especially in the hairline area, can lead to traction alopecia or permanent hair loss due to the damaging effects on the hair follicle. *Note: Braided foundations should not create pain that lasts past the service, or should not be painful to the touch.*

Choosing Hair

Once the method of installation has been considered, choosing the hair is another consideration. Going into a store that sells hair can be overwhelming to a first- timer.

Here are some things to keep in mind when making choices about hair:

Synthetic hair is the most inexpensive, but lacks sustainability. Because it is made of an array of synthetic or man-made fibers, it is not easily passed off as human hair. Synthetic hair is often difficult to flow in the same manner as human hair. Synthetic hair is unable to withstand heat, causing it to melt and disintegrate; and it tangles easily.

Hair that is labeled **Human hair** is often 100% human or mixed with natural fibers, like animal hair. This hair is durable and can be treated like human hair. It is suitable for heated tools, shampooing and styling. Although coloring this hair is possible, it is not advised because the hair has already been chemically treatment to obtain its color and texture. To add more chemicals would damage the hair rendering it dry and tangled; and the coloring process is unpredictable.

Virgin hair or **Cuticle Hair** is the highest quality and offers the most versatility and durability. A bundle will start at an average cost of $80 but can dramatically increase depending on the quality. Virgin hair has not been chemically treated and comes in an array of textures or origins. Therefore, it is better suited for custom blended coloring.

Color. Hair can be purchased in a wide array of colors. Most hair manufacturers use a standard numbering system for levels of color. 1-Black, 4- Medium Brown and 10-Lightest Blonde. When larger numbers are used it usually indicates the multiple colors were used to create a highlight/ lowlight look. Each manufacturer colors will vary and color and most of them will have their own special color blend.

Maintenance Tips

Once you have the hair installed, follow these maintenance tips to keep tresses looking great:

♥ Shampoo regularly. Although shampooing does loosen the braids a bit, it is good for your hair underneath and it keeps the hair flowing and bouncy. Dry shampoo is also an option for keeping the hair clean and free of debris.

♥ It is not a good idea to try and tighten braids. When braids grow out, to avoid breakage remove the extensions and re-install.

♥ Wrap your hair at night and either put on a silk or satin scarf or sleep on a silk or satin pillowcase. Doing this helps the hair to retain its luster and also prevents tangling.

♥ Because the installed hair is often chemically or color treated, a sulfate free shampoo is preferable.

♥It is recommended that excessive heat is not used on the hair. Although hair labeled as "100% human hair" can sustain heat, excessive heat shortens the lifespan of the hair.

♥Don't try to stretch installs past the recommended time. Avoid the temptation to overload the hair with products.

♥When you shampoo hair that is done via a braided install, make sure the braids at the scalp dry completely. If the hair doesn't dry, the hair will mildew and smell.

Extensions are a fun alternative to mundane styling, but must be cared for with caution. Failure to follow the necessary precautions can turn your dream weave to a horrible nightmare. Extreme tension or wearing extension installs past their recommended periods can cause pulling or breakage of the hair and unnecessary discomfort or damage to the scalp.

The lifespan of each install method varies with technique, but should be regarded as a priority when considering which method is best for you. *Braided installs* boast a lifespan of up to 10 weeks, but can cause extreme hair loss if worn too long or not removed properly. After a period of about 12 weeks, coarser hair textures begin to encase itself creating matted locks at the scalp.

Upon removal, be sure to detangle hair thoroughly prior to shampooing, or adding any type of chemical product. Improper detangling is the most common cause for trouble when removing the installations. If not removed with the proper lubricant or removal solutions *braid-less installation* methods such as fusion installs, micro-linking or bonded-in wefts can lead to painful and dangerous removal services. Seeking a professional who is learned in healthy practices will prevent unsafe sessions or irreversible damage. ♥~AT

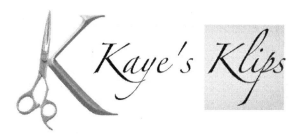

Each year, more than 1000 tons of human hair is imported to the U.S. to accommodate the seemingly infinite demands for weaving and extensions. Twenty five percent of that supply comes from India. From a country where 85% of the people practice Hinduism

and shaving one's head is a common ritual to show humility, the

supply is plentiful.[12]

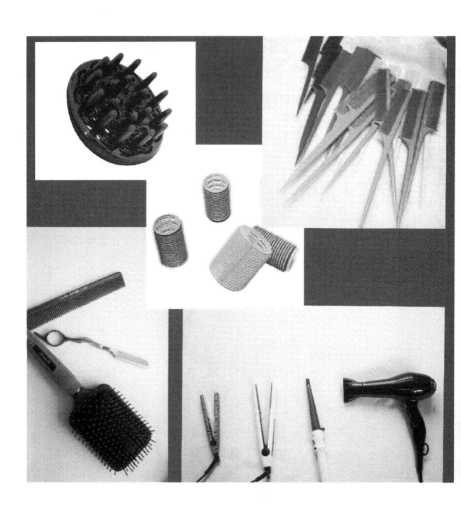

Chapter X
The Mane Tools!

I love when I finish a client's hair and they say, "It doesn't look like this when I do it at home." The most common presumption is that I am applying a product that they are not using. They ask me about every product I use and I tell them. Their next focus is placed on the tools I use.

Getting the best tools does not mean you will get best results because *your capabilities* dictate the outcome. However, a professional in any occupation will attest that you need tools adequate for your job. No matter how good you are at your work, it's extremely difficult to experience continued success with bad tools. Better tools improve productivity and add value to the finished product.

Some people are fond of trying whatever is new. The same is true for tools and products. This can be a good thing because you are open to the new discoveries and find tools that make your life easier. However, the trial and error of this exploration can make or break your hair - yes, pun intended!

For some, sifting through countless types and brands of flat irons trying to figure out which is the best for their hair is not only a headache, but it is absolutely confusing. This is true especially when you actually find several tools that have similar functionalities, but differ drastically in cost. How can you decide which one will work for you without trying them all or having to break the bank?

Many tools; flat irons, blow dryers, curling irons, etc., are labeled "For Professional Use Only." Have you ever wondered what makes a tool "For Professional Use?" Usually it's the quality. Let's look at some of the most common tools, how to use them and when we use them.

Combs

A comb is a comb, is a comb, right? Wrong! Not all combs are created equal, yet many of us just grab the first one we can find. Because the comb is the most fundamental element of hairstyling, using a good quality comb is very important. Combs can be either machine or handmade and made of different materials, and the bristles of different fibers.

The stronger or more durable the fiber, the better the product. A comb that has been molded fairs better because machine made combs or the ones with seams often have little bits of plastic that can snap, pull or tangle the hair. Soft plastic combs are the most inexpensive yet give you less control. Thus, hard plastic combs, even though more expensive, are a stylist's favorite.

You can find lots of combs and variations in a multitude of shapes and sizes, yet here are a few combs and how to use them. Look at the photo from left to right, then the top, and review this list of the most common combs used and their purpose:

1. **All purpose-fork tip:** This comb is great for styling and lifting.

2. **Two-way styling comb:** Designed for lifting or giving the appearance of layering.

3. **Wide-tooth or Shampoo comb:** This is good for combing products, usually conditioner, through the hair.

4. **All-purpose comb:** Multi-use comb; useful for styling, cutting, and molding or setting hair.

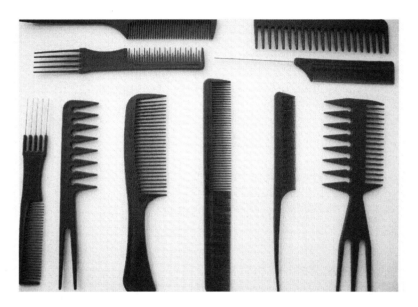

5. **Fine-tooth tail comb or rat-tail comb:** Tail combs are optimal for sectioning and parting the hair. The fine-teeth allow for a smoother finish.

6. **3-way styling comb:** Considered the ultimate styling comb; designed to lift, smooth or add texture.

7. **Wide-tooth tail comb:** Tail combs are optimal for sectioning and parting the hair. The wide-teeth are better suited for coarser hair and offer more control of the hair.

8. **Teasing comb:** Designed for backcombing, or adding cushion to a hairstyle.

9. **Wide-tooth comb:** Excellent for detangling hair.

10. **Metal tip tail comb:** Ideal for parting, lifting or smoothing.

As a rule, fine-toothed combs are designed to create a smooth finish and combs with wide teeth are designed to create a more textured finish.

Note: Discard combs that have broken or missing teeth, as they will pull or break the hair.

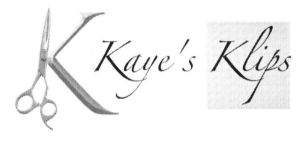 *Did you know that your hairbrush and comb are a breeding ground for germs? Clean them often. Remove all visible signs of hair; use a cleansing shampoo to help remove all build-up. Next, soak them in a mix of hot water that is infused with a few drops of antiseptic.*

This method goes a lot away in preventing scalp infections.

Brushes

Since ancient times, the idea of brushing your hair 100 strokes daily has been perpetuated as a way to promote hair growth and beautiful shiny hair. It is true that stimulation promotes blood circulation, which is a vital for a healthy scalp.

Brushing your hair is important; however, the "100 strokes a day" is not recommended. One of the reasons this practice has changed over the years has to do with the increased amount of stress we put on our hair with chemicals and heated tools; as well as the increased care we give to our hair.

Proper brushing is still a part of routine maintenance; but how and when you should brush depends on the type of hair you have. Extremely wavy or curly hair is best not brushed when trying to maintain the curl pattern. If you choose to blow dry curly hair, use a wide-tooth comb first to untangle the hair before brushing. Never brush wet hair.

Brushing helps to distribute natural oils through the hair. It loosens dead skin cells and dirt and promotes circulation. If your scalp is really dry, using a moisturizer on the scalp and then taking a soft bristle brush; helps get rid of dry skin.

The following picture from left to right shows a few brushes coupled with some uses:

1. **Paddle brush:** The air-filled rubber cushion is designed to bend with your scalp to minimize damage from pulling; ideal for detangling.
2. **Vent brush:** The built-in holes allow air from a blow dryer to flow through to cut drying time and to add volume.
3. **Styling Vent Brush:** allows for air to flow through for faster styling and drying, which offering styling ability.
4. **Small Blow Drying Brush:** Round brushes make it easier to control tension and create a smooth finish when drying.
5. **Large Round Brush:** Great for blow-drying long hair, while adding curl or volume.
6. **Medium Round Brush:** Great for blow-drying medium length hair, while adding curl or volume.
7. **Small Round Brush:** Great for blow-drying short hair, while adding curl or volume.

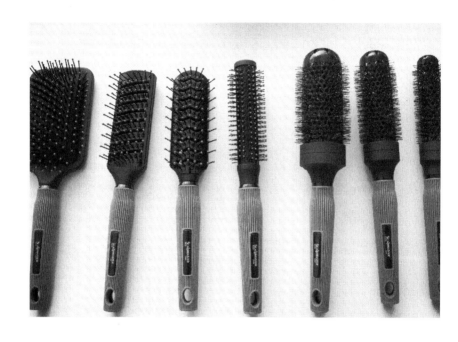

"The worst form of inequality is to try to make unequal things equal." ~*Aristotle*

Types Of Bristles

Although brushes vary in uses, the premier factor that creates a divide between brushes is the type of bristle. A number of bristle patterns are available and they're used for different purposes and hair types. Improve your efforts by buying brushes that work for, instead of against, your *Mane Attraction*.

Boar

This bristle is the actual hair of a boar (hog). Boar bristles are easier on hair than plastic bristles. Boar bristles are considered ideal because they redistribute oils throughout hair, close the cuticle layer and create shiny hair. They are natural, soft and flexible bristles that gently brush the hair. These bristles are suitable for use on children, or persons with fine to normal hair.

Mixed Bristle

Natural bristles alone can be too weak for thicker hair, or to brush through tangles. Mixed bristles, also called porcupine bristles, tend to be stronger because they use a combination of boar and nylon bristles. Mixed bristle brushes are gentle yet exert a good hold on the hair. This brush is an exemplary design for medium to thick hair and for brushing thick hair right down to the scalp.

Nylon/Synthetic

The term synthetic refers to manmade fibers. In context, it refers to bristles made of plastic, nylon, rubber or similar materials. Nylon bristles are the most versatile, ranging from soft and flexible to firm and stiff. Although they can provide a great amount of control for the hair, and some shine; synthetic bristles are non-absorbent and don't distribute natural oils like natural bristles.

Note: As a rule, the stiffer and more closely spaced the bristle, the more control you have over the hair.

Metal

Metal brushes are sometimes used to create height or to finish a style. I recommend them only for styling wigs, or on use of commercial hair. **Metal brushes should never be used on wet hair!** Metal bristles — even with soft plastic tips — are too strong for human hair; they rip the hair and fray the cuticle.

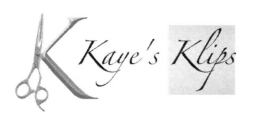

Bristle brushes need to be broken in. The more you use bristle brushes, the more you break them in, making the brush more comfortable and functional.

Heated Tools

Heated tools can be used to create or remove texture. Curling irons and hot rollers are used *to create* a wave or curl; flat irons and blow dryers can be used *to remove* waves or a curl, yielding the sleekest of styles. Even so, shopping for a new flat iron and blow dryer can be almost as daunting as buying a new car!

Though most heated tools boast numerous "features" that look appealing to consumers, salon quality tools really are different. All of the bells and whistles aren't really necessary, yet some of the features are designed to protect your hair. There are so many things to consider, but paying a little more for a quality tool is a reasonable investment.

Let's take a look a look at some power tools and the buzzwords associated with them:

Blow Dryers

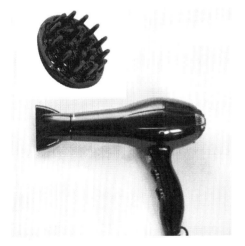

A blow dryer is a handheld electrical device designed to dry hair quickly. The first handheld blow dryer dates back to the 1920's. In the 70's, the soft, carefree blow dry look was popularized by the tresses of Farrah Fawcett. Soon after her rise to stardom, women everywhere wanted the volume, bounce and discipline of her style. Since that time the blow dryer has increased in popularity and solidified its place as a staple in modern day hairstyling and in most American households.

Identifying a blow dryer is not difficult, but selecting one that works best for your needs may be more of a challenge. Is a really expensive hair dryer really better than an inexpensive hair dryer? And what do those terms like "ionic" and "far infrared" really mean?

These are some things you should know when selecting a blow dryer:

Wattage does not indicate heating capacity; it only indicates your hair dryer's power. The three main functions that work together in a hair dryer to determine its quality are airflow (wattage), heat and technology.

Wattage is based on how strong the motor is. The stronger the motor, the higher the watts needed. A smaller motor will have a good lifespan for home usage, and a larger motor is a must for stylists who plan to use the dryer a lot throughout a day. The larger motor makes for a longer lifespan.

Note: Dual voltage dryers convert from 110/120 V to 220/240 V with a standard adapter and then work almost anywhere in the world.

Heating elements. Blow dryers that have metallic or plastic heating parts are less expensive, yet they tend to burn with extremely high heat because essentially they boil the water off of your hair. Coupled with this intense heat, metallic or plastic heating elements tend to heat your hair unevenly. These inexpensive dryers causes positive ions to be left in the hair; which opens the cuticle layer of the hair, leaving the hair frizzy and dull.

In Chemistry 101 you learned that when positive and negative ions are balanced, they are neutralized. Positive ions are created by extreme friction. So anytime you combine the heat of a blow dryer to brushing or combing hair, you create positive ions. **Ionic hair dryers** create negative ions that neutralize hair's positive charge created by the process of drying. The balancing of ions allows the cuticle to remain flat, "trapping" moisture, eliminating frizz and giving hair more body. Ionic hair dryers are able to dry hair faster than regular dryers and leave it shinier and smoother. They are able to do this because they don't "cook" your hair dry like the old metal or plastic coils did – instead, they actually break down water molecules in your hair. Another major benefit of ionic dryers is that they banish the static electricity and resulting flyways that are common in the cheaper heating elements.

Technology

Ceramic

Ceramic materials possess remarkable properties of heat conduction - which you may be familiar with, because modern space heaters and similar home technologies tend to use ceramic. Ceramic is a material that has unique heat conduction properties, resulting in heat that radiates evenly across your hair. Ceramic, which can be infused with tourmaline or other elements, produces a gentle heat that means ceramic heating is safer - ceramic space heaters won't catch things on fire the way metal ones are prone to do, and ceramic hair dryers won't blast your hair with harmful energy.

Infrared

Infrared technology (also called "far-infrared") is a heating method that delivers consistent heat that dries hair evenly and thoroughly. One of the unique qualities of Far-Infrared heat is that it heats from inside the hair follicle to the outside. This protects the surface of the hair and prevents sections of your hair from getting overheated or drying out, resulting in healthier, shinier hair.

Tourmaline

Tourmaline was recently introduced to the hair sciences because of its incredible capability to emit negative ions. Tourmaline is a semi-precious gemstone and is said to be the world's best ionic and infrared generator. When heated, the negative ions generated by the tourmaline splits large water droplets into smaller molecules that immediately evaporate. This dries hair quicker, prevents damage and seals in moisture, resulting in a sleek and shiny finish.

Weight

Select one that best suits your hand. If you're going to use this tool often, it is important to select one that is lightweight and a good fit ergonomically. Professional grade hair dryers tend to be very light because they are designed to be held and used all day long. Some manufacturers even offer featherweight dryers for stylists. A lighter blow dryer will be more comfortable to use even if you're only drying your hair after you get out of the shower.

Settings

A hair dryer with multiple speed settings is standard on professional hair dryers, but they are a nice feature for dryers designed for home use. This feature allows you to customize the heat and airflow depending on your needs. The lower settings are good for styling hair and the higher settings are for more powerful drying. Lower settings are safest for fine or thin hair. "Cool Shot" options available on most hair dryers create a blast of cool air which sets the look for longer lasting hold and adds a shine.

Nozzle or Concentrator

The nozzle or concentrator helps to keep the airflow stream concentrated and directional. This is great if you like to blow-dry your hair straight using a brush.

Diffuser

A diffuser is an optional blow dryer attachment that softens or diffuses the airflow. This is great for drying curly hair to prevent from disturbing the curl pattern; or for lightly drying finishing sprays or hair that has been molded or set in place.

Swivel Cord

A swivel cord at the end of the hair dryer handle allows the electrical cord to pivot and prevents the cord from tangling. This feature is obviously not a crucial feature, rather a luxury feature for professional stylists.

Note: The air intake at the back of the dryer allows air to flow freely. Dirt and hair buildup in the airflow hinders the passage of air, causing the heating element to burn out prematurely.

Flat Irons

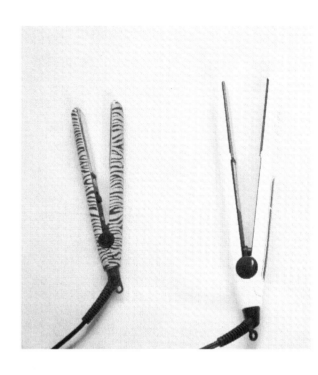

I fearlessly face frizzy flyaway hair armed with a flat iron. It is my favorite styling tool and I feel so empowered with one. There is no greater tool for creating a sleek, polished look than a flat iron. Composed of two flat, heated plates that hinge together to smooth and straighten unruly hairs; a flat iron is relatively easy to use. As simple as it sounds, choosing one is not always as simple. Recently I attended a hair show and in a matter of minutes I saw countless manufacturers selling flat irons, and all claimed to be the best. One thing is sure; there are plenty to choose from; ranging in price from $20 to $200.

Although companies use a slew of clever buzzwords to sell products, three basic considerations are important to focus on when shopping for flat irons: Plate size, plate material and temperature.

Plate Size

Flat irons range in sizes from 1/2 inch to 2 inches. The smaller ones are obviously ideal for shorter hair or getting in tight spaces. Respectively, the 2-inch plates are more appropriate for long hair. If your hair is medium length or if you change your look often, a 1-inch plate is best.

Plate Material

Ceramic: See above.

Tourmaline: See above.

Titanium: Titanium has a very smooth finish, heats up quickly and maintains temperature. It provides intense heat (up to 450° F; hair starts to decompose at temperatures of 410° for fine hair). Titanium is good for thick, coarse or hard to straighten hair. It is also recommended for use in applying keratin treatments. Because of its intense heat, Titanium is not recommended for at home use. Excessive heat will burn hair and lead to breakage.

Silver: This technology eliminates bacteria on the iron plates and your hair, creating a germ-free environment with every use.

Aluminum: Some older, lesser quality flat irons are pure aluminum. These irons are usually referred to as the "drugstore variety" and do not include any of the newer technology; this accounts for the large price disparity in flat irons.

Nano: Whenever you see Nano, think teeny, tiny pieces. Typically, Nano works with other technologies such as Nano Silver or Nano Titanium.

The designation of Nano indicates that micro particles of Silver or Titanium have been infused into the plate. The purpose of the infusion is to enhance the smoothness of the plates allowing them to slide through the strands.

Temperature

The heat in irons is controlled by a microchip that regulates the length of time it takes to reach desired temperatures. Positive Temperature Coefficient (PTC) heaters are the more common heating elements, but they take about two minutes to heat up and the temperature can't be adjusted.

Metal Ceramic Heaters (MCH) utilizes advanced ceramic technology which allows it to reach its desired temperature in five seconds; it is energy efficient, a more reliable heat and the temperature can be adjusted.

If your straightener will be used on more than one type of hair, avoid purchasing a flat iron that does not have an adjustable temperature. You will need to adjust the temperature adequately to straighten different types of hair.

A good rule of thumb: The thicker and wavier the hair, the higher the temperature needed to straighten it.

Recommendations

A quality flat iron works quickly, damages hair less and gives strands a smooth, shiny finish. Because of the technology utilized, a good straightener doesn't have to be the most expensive, but definitely are not the cheapest. Bad flat irons are inefficient and leave your hair a frizzy, damaged mess.

Ceramic and Tourmaline flat irons with MCH heaters are ideal for all hair types and textures. Titanium is better for thicker, coarser and hard to straighten hair.

Curling Irons/Wands/Wavers

Curling irons have been a must in our cosmetic kits for years with no major adjustments to its functionality. But today a demand for curls is on the rise. From slightly tossed beach waves, to tightly coiled, curls comes in a variety of sizes and patterns.

Whether your hair is bone straight and you want to add curls or you want to enhance the ones you have, there's a tool that will do it for you. From barrel curls to spiral curls and everything in between; there is no limit on the looks you can create.

When choosing a curling iron, the basic considerations are: Barrel size, handles, technology and functionality.

Continue reading to learn more about curling irons, and how to choose them:

Barrel Size

The barrel is the most important aspect of determining the size and shape of your curl. Determining the best barrel size depends on the length of your hair and the desired style. Obviously, the bigger the barrel size the bigger the curl.

Before purchasing a curling iron, you must carefully consider what you want the irons to accomplish; doing this will guide you in determining the size. Barrels range in size from 1/8-inch which offers a tiny pencil curl to 2-inches which offers more of a loose wave.

If you change your length and style often, several barrel sizes may be needed. An alternative which offers more variety is to buy a curling iron offering interchangeable barrels.

Handles

Marcel: The Marcel® iron has the extra handle. This iron renders the most control in styling; when used properly this iron produces the best curl. However, it is designed for professionals and is the most difficult to master. If you are not skilled at using this iron, your best option is to select a different one. If you have a Marcel® iron, be sure to practice manipulating them while they are cold.

Spring Clip: As the name suggests, these irons have the spring clip handle, instead of the long handle featured on the Marcel® iron. A spring clip offers ease in styling and a firm hold.

The spring clip handle is the easiest to use and the preferred type of handle for the consumer. With this iron no manipulation s of the fingers required; the thumb only is employed to catch and release the curls.

Clip-less: In the clip-less iron, no clip is used to hold the hair in place while curling. This iron takes some getting used to, but it definitely has its benefits. The hair is wrapped around the iron and briefly held for curl formation.

Most clip-less irons come with a heat resistant glove to protect your hand and fingers. With the elimination of the clip, the irons are able to get closer to the scalp; and offer smoother curls with no creases.

Technology

Much of the technology used in heated tools transcends from implement to implement. To understand more about the technology used in curling irons, refer to the section on flat irons.

Functionality

Most irons are flexible and can create several curl patterns. However, there are more specific irons that function better for specific looks, but they are good for that one look only. For example, a crimping iron makes more uniformed crimps than curling irons, but they are only good for producing crimps.

Care and Maintenance

To keep the irons at optimal performance, wipe the irons off after each use to remove dirt, oils or any product residue.

The tools we use are essential to creating and maintaining a flawless mane. While they don't possess any super powers, using the wrong tools can wreak havoc on your hair. Your hair will be with you for a while, at least we hope so; it's better to make an investment in quality tools.

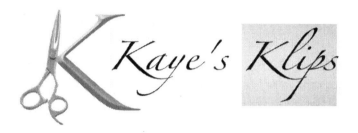

Marcel® irons are named for Francois Marcel, a 19th century French hairdresser who invented the process of marcel waving in 1872. This processed revolutionized the art of hairdressing all over the world and remained in vogue for over 50 years.

The original irons were heavy tongs that were heated over a gas burner. As you can imagine, with such primitive equipment it was hard to maintain the correct temperature for the iron - too cool and the wave did not set, too hot and the hair got burnt. The hairdresser tested the iron on a piece of paper before using it on a client's hair. If the paper burnt, the iron was too hot! In 1924 electric waving irons were available for which the temperature of the iron could be regulated.[13]

Just Ask Faye

Chapter VI
Answering Your Questions And
Debunking The Myths

What is dandruff? What is the difference between breakage and shedding? These are questions that I hear regularly and I love to answer those queries. But, I have heard many erroneous fables that promise to return hair to a majestic luster: Boil a cup of mustard oil with four tablespoons of henna leaves, let it cool, and then massage it daily onto the balding areas for hair loss reversal. Even better; cutting your hair on a full moon will make hair grow back longer and more voluminous. The worst: Cow feces and pig urine are both good topical solutions to ward off balding.

Sound crazy? Well, of course . . . Sadly, there are some who are so desperate for an antidote to their hair dilemmas that they are willing to give *anything* a try. We often hear old wives' tales that have been passed down from generation to generation. When it comes to hair care, a lot of information is out there; some reasonable and some that is completely lunatic.

Even in the Information Age, misinformation always abounds and can prove extremely harmful to your hair. (By the way, everything on the Internet is not true). I have compiled a list of questions that I am often asked often and myths that I have heard perpetuated. Let's answer those questions and shed some light on these myths!

Answering Your Questions

What is dandruff?

Dandruff is a shedding of the skin on the scalp that leaves white flakes on the head, neck and shoulders. It may also be a form of a skin condition called eczema, which causes increased shedding of normal scalp skin cells. Dandruff can also be caused by a fungal infection.

What is psoriasis? (Response contributed by Rodney Barnett)

Psoriasis is characterized by patches of red skin covered by silvery-white scales that are present on the elbows, knees and scalp. No one knows the cause of psoriasis, but it comes about because of abnormal cell division. Normal skin cells have a life span of about 28 days. With psoriasis the skin cells turn over at a rate 10 times faster than normal cells, causing a build-up of scales in thick, red and scaly patches. Psoriasis is often precipitated or aggravated by physical or emotional stress, upper respiratory infections, strep throat, alcoholic beverages, obesity, certain oral medications (lithium and anti-malarial drugs), and skin injuries such as scratches, cuts, and burns that include sunburns. This chronic skin disease causes some itching but does not cause hair loss.

What is seborrhea dermatitis?

Seborrhea dermatitis is a common, chronic inflammatory skin disorder. The condition is not harmful or contagious, but it can be uncomfortable and unsightly. It is characterized by redness and scaling.

On the scalp seborrhea dermatitis can range from a mild case of dandruff to thickened scaling patches and may pose an itching sensation. It often spreads to the face or other area of the skin that have very active sebaceous glands. On the face it appears as powdery or greasy scales showing up in the creases around the nose, the forehead, the inner eyebrows and the external ear canal. The upper eyelids and eyelid margins may also be involved.

Seborrhea dermatitis is triggered by stress, fatigue and change of season; with the winter being the worst.

How fast should my hair grow?

Hair grows about 1/2 inch a month in a healthy adult. Hair grows faster in for youth 18-22 and grows more slowly as you age.

What is the difference between shedding and breakage?

Shedding is long strand hair loss or hair that comes from the scalp. Shedding is most often a result of something internal like medicines, diet or the natural growth and loss process.

Breakage is short strand hair loss. It is usually the result of chemical process, and indicates that the hair was in some way compromised, and it broke. Dry, brittle, over processed hair is more prone to breakage.

What is alopecia?

Alopecia is hair loss or balding. There are several types of alopecia.

Alopecia areata is "area" hair loss or hair loss that occurs in totally smooth round patches. This usually occurs as a result of an autoimmune disease, allergies or eczema. In some cases alopecia areata can be as a result of taking medications. Hair loss resulting from alopecia areata usually grows back in six months to a year.

Traction alopecia is hair loss that is caused by extreme tension, pulling or friction; usually in the case of tight ponytails, braids or hair extensions. If the tension is removed the hair often grows back. If the localized trauma is persistent or prolonged the result is often scalp damage and permanent hair loss.

Scarring alopecia is hair loss that is caused by an inflammatory condition like burns, injury or bacterial infection.

Androgenic alopecia/Male Pattern Baldness (MPB) is hormonal hair loss that occurs as a result of the loss of androgens. Androgens are called "male" hormones, but are present in both men and women. Since our hormones should operate in harmony, an imbalance will cause problems; hair loss is one. MPB is the most common type of balding occurring in 70% of men and 40% of women.

Diffused alopecia is a type of androgenic alopecia in which the balding is more diffused or thin. Diffused alopecia is more common in women and is therefore called Female Pattern Balding (FPB).

Telogen Effluvium (TE) is a type of hair loss associated with traumatic or stressful events. Ninety percent of your hair strands typically are in the anagen or growing phase. After a stressful event, more of the hair shifts to the telegen or resting phase, causing the hair to shed. This shedding takes places usually about six weeks after the stressful event. The hair will soon return to the growing phase after the stress subsides.

How often should I shampoo?

You should shampoo as often as you need to. Some hair types are excessively oily and should be shampooed more often than person with extremely dry hair. Shampooing weekly is a good idea for all hair types. When you shampoo be sure to condition to replenish the moisture.

How often should I have my ends trimmed?

Usually every six-to-eight weeks is sufficient.

Can I use a good conditioner to mend split ends?

No, because once hair grows from the root, hair is not alive and it is not possible to "heal" the hair. Practicing good hair maintenance is best to prevent split ends, but once ends are split, trimming them is the only cure.

How do I remove upper lip hair without shaving?

There are several options to upper lip and chin hair removal. If you are removing only a few stray hairs, *tweezing* is the best option. When removing more hair, this process can be more painful.

Waxing is another quick and easy solution. There is a slight risk of irritation from the wax, but it is effective (although not permanent).

A *depilatory* is another quick method that is pain free. The chemicals involved are harsh so it's important to select a depilatory made especially for delicate skin.

Threading, much like waxing, is another quick and easy solution. This process can be painful, yet it is effective (but not permanent).

Electrolysis or laser hair removal offer more permanent solutions, but both require several treatments and can be costly. Electrolysis is laborious and uses a tiny needle inserted into each hair follicle to destroy it. Laser hair removal requires fewer treatments but is more costly. This process involves using a laser to zap the hair at the root to permanently destroy the follicle. Careful research should be given when choosing a hair removal specialist.

What is a depilatory and how does it work?

A **depilatory** is a hair removal crème designed to eliminate unwanted hair. Depilatories are alkaline-based products with an extremely high pH and designed to decompose unwanted hair. As the hair decomposes, simply wipe off and rinse with warm water. Although the process is quick and easy, it often comes with a pungent odor and can cause some skin irritation.

How do I go from a high lift blonde back to a dark brunette or black without turning "funky" green?

Going from a really light color to a really dark color can be challenging. Most people find that their color fades easily or has a translucent look. To avoid this, you must apply a filler. A *protein filler* helps equalize the porosity of the hair and gets into the gaps of the cuticle so that the hair color penetrates evenly. A *color filler* adds color back into the hair. Usually a color filler adds one of the primary colors; red, blue or yellow back into the hair.

Does haircolor change my natural texture?

As much as I love color, haircolor can be harsh and drying, especially haircolor that requires bleaching. Hair that is already dry and fragile can lose its natural curl pattern. But conditioning the hair before and after color will help the hair to maintain its integrity.

How can I keep my permanent red color from fading?

A good, long-lasting red color is sometimes difficult to manage. Red haircolor is usually the fastest to fade. However, permanent haircolor generally is permanent, but does get dulled down by frequent shampooing. Red haircolor is a high maintenance color because it requires frequent refreshers. It is important to seal the haircolor with a conditioning color sealant to help maintain the color.

When can I expect to go grey?

There is no specific age when grey appears. To have a better idea of when you might grey, look at both your parents and see when they greyed; it is likely you will follow one of them.

Why is my grey hair so stubborn?

As hair greys it not only loses its pigment, the cuticle also tightens, thus making it more difficult for products and moisture to penetrate the hair.

How young is too young to for chemical straighteners or haircolor?

There is no definitive answer to this question. Several factors should be considered before considering chemicals. First, one should consider the sensitive nature of youthful skin and scalp, and determine if you are willing to apply the harsh chemicals. Also, one should consider if the child is patient enough to endure the process? Sometimes, children are incredibly restless and for these children, sitting still to undergo chemical procedures is difficult. Lastly, a parent should consider the maintenance and upkeep required for the service. Determine if the child is able to handle such responsibility; if not, a parent should be willing to commit to the required level of care.

If I have gastric bypass surgery or a weight loss procedure, will my hair fall out?

Some people experience significant hair loss after weight loss procedures, but the hair loss is not attributed directly to the procedure. Instead, as we discussed before, much of your hair growth has to do with diet. So when you undergo surgery that significantly reduces the intake of nutrients, or if you go on diets that eliminate whole categories of food, taking vitamins or a supplement to replace those lost nutrients becomes very important.

Is there something I can take to make my hair grow thicker?

The density of your hair is determined by genetics. There is no magic pill that can change genetics and make your hair denser. However, if your hair was fuller and is thinning due to over-processing or circumstantial causes, a multi-vitamin and a healthy diet rich in vitamins and antioxidants will nurture hair growth.

What is a keratin straightener?

Keratin is a protein that is naturally in your hair. A keratin straightener is more of a restorative treatment that puts keratin back in the hair. It works by applying a keratin hair-straightening product to your hair and then using the heat of a flat iron to seal in the product. In order to help the keratin penetrate the cuticle, manufacturers once used formaldehyde to open the cuticle.

After concerns raised by the Federal Drug Administration, companies began manufacturing keratin straighteners without formaldehyde.

Can I perm or color hair extensions?

Many hair manufacturers apply chemical treatments to hair extensions during the production phase to add texture and color. If this production technique occurs with the extensions you purchased, adding *more* chemicals would be disastrous. The level of manipulation possible with your hair extensions depends on the quality of extensions you purchased. In order to be able to perm the hair extensions, they need to be human hair extensions that were not chemically treated prior to purchase.

I am extremely tender headed! What causes me to be so tender headed? Is there anything I can take to ease the pain?

We all have a different threshold or tolerance for pain and nothing can change our individual threshold. For some, being tender headed is inherent; however, there may be some contributing factors making your scalp tender: Dry skin, tightly tied hair, allergic reactions or fungal infections. If your pain is resulting from one of the contributors, remedy these problems to alleviate the pain. Otherwise, take an over-the-counter pain medicine will help ease the pain.

If a person's hair has matted, is cutting the hair off the only option?

If hair is matted, cutting the hair off is not always a necessity. Removing the matted hair will involve some hair loss, and extreme care must be given to remove tangles without losing excessive hairs.

Using a wide-toothed comb, gently start at the bottom of the matted hair and try to work some of the hairs free from the mass. Remember to exercise patience! If this procedure shows progress, continue as far as you can until the hair is again free and loose. You will need a bottle of detangling spray, leave-in conditioner or maybe something thicker like olive oil. This oil is an added bonus for cases in which the hair is very dry or damaged.

For more tangled masses, you may need to make a cut to loosen the hair a little without removing a lot of the hair.

To do this, take your scissors and direct them toward the scalp. Cut three-quarters of the way through the matted mass directly down the center. Continue working with the wide-tooth comb to loose and free the hairs.

DO NOT MASSAGE OR MANIPULATE. Doing so will cause more matting.

Do we experience hair growth after we die?

This may sound like a ridiculous question to some, but when I was in college I was the hairstylist at a local funeral home. When I finished styling the hair of the deceased, I would often hear bereaved family members say that their loved one's hair appeared longer.

The deceased's hair didn't grow, yet for some people it may appear that the hair has grown longer since the loved one's death. This illusion originates from the dehydration of the dead person's skin, which stretches the skin away from the hair, thus making the hair appear longer in length.

Debunking the Myths

Read through the following "True or False" questions to learn the difference between hair facts and hair fiction:

Trimming your ends will make your hair grow.

False

Hair grows from nutrients in the blood stream. Trimming your ends is a good grooming habit. It makes hair to look nice and polished, but trimming hair doesn't make it grow.

Just as trimming the bushes in front of your house doesn't make the bushes grow any faster, so it is with trimming your ends. Trimming the bushes in front of your house makes your home look more polished and cared for. Don't stop having your ends trimmed; it is a good grooming practice. Just know that it won't make your hair grow back faster.

You can mend split ends with the right products.

False

Split ends are caused when the hair is dry and brittle. It's important to keep your hair moisturized, but the "cure" for split ends is a trim. Conditioners can seal the cuticle of the hair and make the ends less obvious.

Select a conditioner that moisturizes your hair and protects your hair from the heat. A modest trim every 6 to 8 weeks will keep your ends looking good.

You need to eventually switch products so your hair won't "get used" to the same one.

False

If the product is formulated the same, it will always have the same result. However, we are always evolving and changing. Sometimes those changes are manifested in our hair. If your hair changes, you need to switch to a product to meet the needs of your hair.

If the product you're currently using no longer seems to give you the desired result; more than likely you and your hair care needs have changed, not the product.

Brush 100 times a day so hair will grow.

False

Because the hair grows through the circulation of blood, it is a good idea to stimulate the blood circulation to the scalp. Brushing can stimulate circulation but in fact, over-brushing causes friction in the scalp, which can lead to cuticle damage and breakage.

Brush minimally for detangling and styling. Try using a brush with natural bristles or instead use a wide-toothed comb.

You shouldn't shampoo hair too often; this will dry it out.

False

Maintaining a healthy scalp is important. You should shampoo as often as needed. This varies from person to person depending on hair type and lifestyle. Obviously, a person with naturally oily hair or one with a more active lifestyle should shampoo more often. However, one should shampoo at least weekly in order to maintain a healthy scalp. Shampooing may remove some moisture from dry hair, but finding a good moisturizing shampoo and moisturizing conditioner will help to replenish the moisture.

Using washing powder or highly alkaline soaps will strip a permanent wave or chemical relaxer off your hair.

False

Both permanent waves and chemical relaxers permanently alter the hair structure. There is no solution or potion that will reverse the effects of these chemical services. The only way to "change" them will be to cut the chemically treated hair off or wait for it to grow out.

Using washing powder or a highly alkaline shampoo will dry the hair and raise the cuticle. This will make the hair appear rough, as though chemicals are not present. Using these types of products only adds more damage to the hair.

Olive oil or mayonnaise can be used to deep condition your hair.

True

A number of home remedies will work to condition the hair, but don't expect a magic potion. A measure of caution should be used because many home remedies will be extremely heavy and can weigh the hair down. When using these concoctions, use in moderation. Be mindful of the fact that many products are formulated especially for your hair type, reasonably priced, effective and readily available.

Dandruff will help your hair to grow.

False

Dandruff is shedding of the skin on the scalp that leaves white flakes on the head, neck and shoulders. It may be a form of a skin condition called eczema, which causes increased shedding of normal scalp skin cells. Dandruff can also be caused by a fungal infection. Hormonal or seasonal changes can make dandruff worse.

Dandruff definitely doesn't cause hair to grow; as a matter of fact, in extreme cases when the condition is not managed effectively, hair loss can occur as a by-product of this situation. Shampoos and conditioners containing zinc pyrithione are the most effective remedy for dandruff since they prevent re-growth of the fungus, thus acting as a preventative measure for both dandruff and the hair loss linked to scratching.

Coloring/dyeing your hair while pregnant is harmful to the fetus.

False

The Organization of Teratology Information Services (OTIS), an organization which provides information on potential reproductive risks, says that there is little to no potential risk of haircolor being absorbed in the bloodstream to cause damage. Years ago many color formulations contained excessive amounts of ammonia which were often ingested in the lungs and could be harmful to the baby. Today many formulations have much less ammonia. Just make sure the area where the color is applied is well ventilated.[13]

This is an important time for you and your baby, if you are still concerned, consider waiting to the second trimester to add color and speak to your doctor.

Exposure to sunlight is the healthiest way to lighten your hair color.

False

A significant amount of sun is required to start lightening hair. Your scalp is a very sensitive place and can get sunburned without you even knowing. Exposure to harsh sunlight will raise the pH of the hair and swell the cuticle, which can dry out the hair follicles and leave your hair feeling brittle.

The chemicals used in most hair lightening products are very safe and easy to use. Always follow excessive sun exposure with a conditioning treatment to balance the pH balance of your hair.

Sulfur 8® or Glover's Mane® (Dog Mane) will make your hair grow.

False

This idea was first introduced in the early 1900's in Madame CJ Walker's miracle hair grower, where she used therapeutic sulfur for hair growth. It was extremely helpful in its era, because her products were marketed to Black women, who at that time very rarely were able to shampoo their hair. When they did, most often they would use leftover dish or bath water that was highly contaminated with bacteria. As a result these women had very unhealthy scalps that led to hair loss. The sulfur helped to heal the scalp creating an environment more conducive for hair growth.[14]

Now that we have more improved hygiene habits for our hair, a sulfur regimen is not needed.

Greasing your hair or scalp will help hair to grow.

False

The goal for all hair is to find a moisture balance. So for hair that is excessively oily the object is to remove some of the oil.

By contrast, hair that is excessively dry needs moisture. Hair grease can be a source of moisture. However, this moisture will not help hair grow; it protects the hair and keeps it from breaking.

If you choose to use hair or scalp oil, use it sparingly because excessive amounts will not only weigh the hair down, using too much of this product can clog the hair follicles and impede growth.

If you pluck out one grey hair, two or three will sprout in its place.

False

Plucking out grey hair does not create more grey hair, however, this practice is not encouraged. The hair will grow back unless the follicle is damaged, and it will still be grey when it returns. Plucking hair creates scalp irritation which can be harmful to the hair follicle.

If you start to see grey hairs, try a color that is especially formulated for grey coverage or use a hair mascara product until you are able to get it colored.

Stress makes your hair turn grey.

True and False

The timing of your hair turning grey and the amount of hair that turns grey is primarily determined by your genes. A little stress, such as the stress of meeting a deadline, or driving in evening traffic do not contribute to excessive amounts of stress. However, severe and chronic stress that causes physiological changes in the body will accelerate the greying process.

It should be noted that illness, sudden and traumatic loss of a loved one or the extreme stress associated with an office as significant as that of President of the United States does cause levels of stress that can accelerate the greying process.

You should always shampoo your hair with cold water.

False

Actually shampooing with warm water is better because doing so helps to open the cuticle and remove build-up from hair. Shampooing with warm water is also effective in removing dirt and debris from the hair.

Rinsing with *cool* water (*not cold*) is also not a bad idea, particularly for color- treated hair. Hair cuticles, which resemble shingles on a roof, lie flat when splashed with cool water. As a result, the smoothed cuticles reflect more light, making hair appear shinier and healthier. The effect is temporary if not followed with a product like a leave-in conditioner that will add shine.

Hair should not be shampooed with hot water. Not only is it uncomfortable, doing so it leaves hair rough and lackluster.

Natural shampoos are the only ones that are gentle enough for colored or chemically treated hair.

False

The hair industry has certainly excelled and manufacturers have noted that consumers want gentler options. Lots of shampoos are on the market; many are sulfate free and they contain natural oils, which have been proven to be gentle enough not to weaken the hair.

It's normal for hair to shed.

True

Hair sheds an average of 50 to 100 strands a day. This shedding should not be very obvious. Over the course of the day, you will shed a few strands while sleeping, changing clothes, combing hair or even when hair is blowing in the wind.

Anything in excess of the 50-100 daily strands of hair loss is not normal.

Pulling your hair in a ponytail can lead to bald spots.

True

Extreme stress on hair, such as excessive pulling or keeping your hair tightly bound for long periods of time is a leading cause of traction alopecia, which is a type of balding. The constant tension involved in ponytails that are too taut can damage the hair follicle causing hair to stop growing, or lead to some breakage. If the hair follicle is repeatedly subjected to this trauma it can result in permanent hair loss.

Avoid elastic bands with metal and try a smaller band instead of a bulky band. Make the ponytail smooth, but not too tight. *Note: If your ponytail makes you feel like you got an instant facelift, it's too tight!*

Hair grows faster during the summer.

True

Like everything else in nature, summer is a time of productivity. Hair grows from the nutrients in the blood stream. Because we tend to be more active in the warmer weather, and because the warm weather helps in circulation; hair grows faster. Also, sun exposure helps the body with Vitamin D consumption, which is an essential element in the hair growth cycle.

Male-Pattern Baldness is passed down by the mother.

False

MPB is passed genetically, but it is much more complicated than coming from a specific parent. MPB can be inherited from either parent. The balding gene can be inherited by both men and women, but it is usually more pronounced in men.

Stress makes your hair fall out.

True

All of us experience stressful days or situations. However, routine stress is not problematic to hair. On the other hand, life-shattering events like sickness, death of a loved one or divorce often causes telogen effluvium, a form of hair loss that appears randomly across the head as a result of sudden or intense stress. This type of hair loss often occurs two-to-three months after the stressful event. Because the follicles are not harmed, hair loss from telogen effluvium will grow back if the stressful situation is not ongoing.

Cutting a baby's hair before his/her 1st birthday will mess up their hair.

False

Each of us is subject to a change in texture. Most children are not born with the texture they will keep. Shaving a baby's head will not alter the texture of their hair nor will it cause their hair to grow faster or thicker. The biggest concern is finding a stylist that is skilled enough to cut the hair on "a moving target!" The first haircut is usually scary to a child so it is likely he/she will move a lot and possibly even cry.

Chlorine water can change your hair color.

True

It is not uncommon for swimmers with natural blonde or chemically highlighted hair to notice green tints. Because the hair is extremely porous it is absorbing the chlorinated water. To remedy this problem, shampoo the hair with an acid balance shampoo which helps restore the pH of the hair. Also, misting the hair with a leave-in conditioner before entering the pool is also a good idea. Misting the hair with a leave-in conditioner will prevent the absorption of the chlorinated water.

Sleeping with a wet head causes scalp fungus.

False

Scalp or fungal diseases can't be caught from sleeping with wet scalps. Scalp fungus or infections requires prior involvement with infected sources such as humans, tainted hair care tools or animals. As an example, ringworm can be spread by infected animals. However, sleeping with a wet head can cause the hair to sour and produce a very unpleasant odor.

By placing a chemical relaxer mix or no-lye relaxer in the refrigerator you can extend the shelf life.

False

It is ideal to keep all salon chemicals at a moderate room temperature. Relaxers that require mixing (No-Lye) have a shelf life of 24 to 48 hours, after being mixed, depending on the manufacturer. Relaxers that come premixed have a shelf life of one to three years depending on the manufacturers' recommendation. Discard any relaxer once it has exceeded its shelf life because it is unstable and can be very dangerous to the hair. Refrigerating will not extend the product's lifespan.

Do you have a question you would like to ask? Follow me on Twitter @kflewellen, "Like" my Facebook page at Facebook.com/ Just Ask Kaye or contact me via my website at KFlewellen.com.

For all things hair, fashion, beauty and empowerment, Just Ask Kaye™!

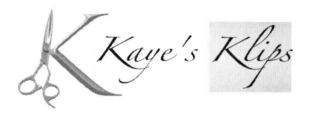

Born Sarah Breedlove, and the daughter of former slaves; Madam C J Walker has secured her place in history as a cosmetology success story. She is often credited with inventing the pressing comb. In addition, she created hair care products, built a factory and a training school. She is also lauded for her "direct sales" marketing strategies, very similar to those used by the Mary Kay® cosmetics company. Madame Walker later became a philanthropist, lobbyist, and political activist; all while organizing the first women's business organization.[15]

Appendix A

Do you need a refresher?

When was the last time you actually sought out a new hairstyle? If it's taking you a while to come up with an answer then it's probably time for a change!

Take this fun quiz and see if your look could use an update. Choose just one answer for each question.

1. Which of these words best describes you?

1. Boring

2. Busy

3. Adventurous

4. Pretty

2. Which of the following best describes your style?

1. Chic and cutting edge

2. Classical

3. Sporty or Dressy, I love both

4. Hard to define

3. Your last new haircut was:

1. Within the past six months

2. Within the past year

3. Within the past two years

4. Within the past five years

4. Your last haircolor application was:

1. Within the past six months

2. Within the past two years

3. More than two years ago

4. More than five years ago; or never

5. What is your bad hair day quick fix?

1. A nice ponytail or bun

2. A baseball cap

3. Tons of gel

4. Every day is a bad hair day!

6. How often do strangers compliment your hair?

1. Very often

2. Regularly

3. Occasionally

4. Never

7. Why do you avoid updating your look?

1. I don't, I love to update!

2. I think I look fine the way I am

3. I don't know where to start

4. I have better things to worry about than how I look

8. Which styling tools do you use the most?

1. Just a comb or brush

2. A flat iron or curling iron

3. A scrunchie or rubber band

4. Whatever I feel like

9. How much time do you spend daily on your hair?

1. Approximately 15 minutes

2. Five - 10 minutes

3. Closer to an hour

4. Less than five minutes

10. What is your ideal hairstyle?

1. The one I wear now

2. One that is popular on celebrities

3. I don't have time for fantasies

4. The one I wore before

Beside each answer there is a number. Add up the number associated with each of your answers to see how you've done.

Results:
30 or above – You are looking good!

20-29 – You are looking good, but a few changes wouldn't hurt.

10-19 – You should consider a refresher.

Below 10 – You need to do something fast – visit a stylist ASAP!

Contributors

SAMI G

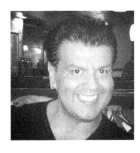

Trendsetter, innovator, global artiste SAMI G. is one of the most sought after colourists of the 21st century. Instructor, master stylist and certified colourist, SAMI G is a leader in the industry with 20+ years of experience working with hair. Educator and Creative Artistic Team Member for global Farouk Inc. for several years, SAMI G has an extraordinary ability to assess a client and determine the most flattering cut, colour and style for their features, skin pigment and personality. SAMI is constantly upgrading his repertoire by continuing education with global masters. HE IS ALWAYS IMITATED BUT NEVER DUPLICATED

SAMI G has been a salon owner for over 25 years. He has been an educator for Scruples, and was one of the original ARTISTIC TEAM MEMBERS for global Farouk Systems. Well-traveled and cultured, SAMI G has performed in every major city in the United States and brought back the latest trends to the Dallas area for over 25 years. He is currently in the works to open his own very private and exclusive beauty school. SAMI G is will have his BBA in Fall 2013 and continue on to his MBA.

Deshonica Kerrie

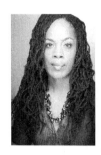

Deshonica Kerrie is a Global Educator as well as a Master Cosmetologist and owner of the Deshonica Kerrie® brand.

Deshonica Kerrie is also a motivational speaker that encourages and acknowledges intrinsic beauty. She has been in the beauty industry since 1992 and has a strong passion for the path that she has chosen.

Deshonica Kerrie also works as a hairstylist on many photo shoots that express her talents and share her work through many publications. She enjoys working as a high fashion hairstylist for fashion shows and being a host for many Natural Hair and Health Expos. She believes understanding healthy hair starts from within so she encourages you to live, laugh, love and have a healthy lifestyle, and encourages maintenance for great results.

Deshonica Kerrie has traveled nationally and internationally educating and helping to connect the professional as well as the client to understand why beauty and education go hand-in- hand.

Jill Waggoner, M.D.

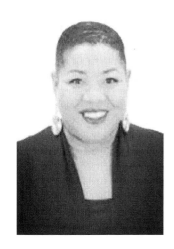

Dr. Jill Waggoner is one of the most sought after medical speakers. She is well known for her unique presentation style which is both educational and entertaining. Affectionately known as "Dr. Jill," she has a unique background in that she was a member of the famed Dallas Cowboys Cheerleaders for three years, and appeared with the group internationally. Dr. Jill holds a Master's Degree and a Medical Degree from the University of Oklahoma. She has certifications in both Preventive Medicine and Wellness Coordination from the Prestigious Cooper Institute. She is a residency trained, board certified Family Practice Physician and has practiced in the Dallas area for more than 18 years. Dr. Jill has a special interest in Integrative Medical, and approaches the treatment of patients from a whole person, total healing perspective.

She is a radio personality and discusses relevant medical topics weekly on the "Ask Dr. Jill" radio segment and "Da Blues" syndicated radio show. She has served as a medical expert for TBN, NBC, and ABC, and is a national medical expert for Fox affiliate radio. Dr. Jill has been a conference speaker for thousands of women including those who have attended the international "Woman Thou Art Loosed" and "Megafest" conference. She is an author who has written for newspapers and magazines including "Emotions." Dr. Jill has penned three books; "My Sister's Keeper, Is Your Temple In Order?," "Stress, Your Secret Weapon" and "Hormone Harmony."

Rodney Barnett

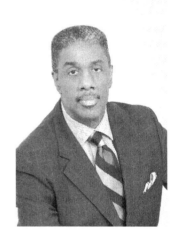

Well-known throughout the country as one of the leading practitioners of Trichology, Rodney Barnett has helped thousands of clients to regain beautiful, lustrous hair. More than that, with his well-attended seminars, he has taught hundreds of licensed cosmetologists to do the same.

Holding a Bachelor of Science degree from the International Institute of Trichology, Huntsville, AL, and a certification from the National Association of Certified Natural Health Professionals, Warsaw, IN, Barnett is a respected expert in the field who has appeared on national television and been quoted extensively in magazines and newspapers throughout the country.

Barnett's method is individual and thorough, beginning with extensive questioning, a microscopic exam and a biochemical assessment. Most importantly, Barnett brings into the equation, the client's diet, exercise and other elements of his or her lifestyle. "All aspects must be considered," he says. "People sometimes want a quick fix, thinking a topical application of a product will solve the problem. If they don't consider all the possible causes, and address them, they won't get to the root, so to speak of the disorder, and even if it is eliminated in the short term, it can easily return."

Available to the press, media and appropriate companies as a spokesperson, Barnett has forged business relationships with medical and naturopathic doctors, dermatologists, nutritionists, herbalists and cosmetologists. He works with them to determine and provide the best solutions for each individual's case and to verify that he stays current with the latest research and treatments. Barnett has been interviewed on ABC's "Good Morning, Texas," CBS's "Positively Texas," Fox's "Insight," and UPN's "City Magazine" among many news programs. He has been quoted in articles in *Essence, Star and Heart & Soul* among other magazines, and has written for several Texas newspapers. Seminars have been recently conducted by Barnett and held throughout the United States and the West Indies.

Rod Warner

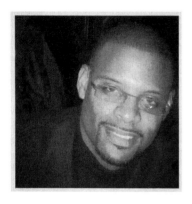

Rod Warner, founder of "Rod Warner Fitness" is a Certified Personal Trainer that provides expert knowledge and coaching to help others reach their fitness goals. Prior to the development of "Rod Warner Fitness," Rod was an educator in the Dallas Independent School District for 10 years. He provided his expertise in the area of Reading and Criminal Justice to students in grades 6-12. Rod was also one of the masterminds behind the Dallas local nightlife magazines titled *In House Magazine* from 2002-2007. Rod graduated from Prairie View A&M University with a Bachelor of Arts Degree in 1998 and a Masters in Counseling in 2008. He also earned a Funeral Science Degree from Dallas Funeral Services in 2008. In 2013 Rod started a non-profit organization, The Rod Warner Foundation, where he mentors young males on health and fitness. Rod met Angela, the love of his life at Prairie View A&M University. They have been married for 15 years and have a beautiful 11-year old daughter named Brooke.

About the Author

Kaye Flewellen is a Baylor University graduate with a Bachelor of Science degree in Communications/Public

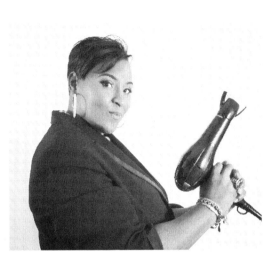

Relations, Salon Owner, Celebrity Stylist, Image Consultant, and Adjunct Professor at Navarro College of Cosmetology. Building on her family's rich history in the hair care industry, her personal studies in cosmetology, trichology, esthetics, and makeup artistry along with more than 20 years of experience, K emerges as a premier voice on all things beauty.

Her passion drives her as a sought after speaker, teacher and mentor.

Kaye has volunteered for several community organizations. In 2008 she became a founding board member of the Rollings

Foundation, an organization focusing on poverty in South Africa. The mission of the Rollings Foundation is to meet the health and educational needs of children by supplying daily lunches and school supplies, planting vegetable gardens and digging water wells. Her work with the Rollings Foundation is one of Kaye's proudest accomplishments. On a mission trip to South Africa in January 2013 Kaye served in the Foundation's soup kitchen and spoke at one of the organization's sponsored orphanages.

In 2010 Kaye entered a partnership with the United States Center for Disease Control (CDC) to educate stylists on AIDS awareness and prevention. Her commitment to HIV awareness also involves serving as host for a free annual HIV testing event in a Dallas community heavily affected by the virus.

Baylor University Alumni Association recently recognized Kaye as a "Distinguished Alumni" for her philanthropic efforts both in her community and abroad.
Having produced styles and articles for national hair magazine publications and worked as a Certified Educator for several hair care companies; Kaye brought her God-given

gifts, writing abilities, business savvy, community service and personal inspiration to one stage. The result: JustAskK.com. Kaye now conveniently avails all of her knowledge and experience via her web space . . . If you have questions regarding all things hair, beauty, fashion, and empowerment, Just Ask K™!

A celebrity stylist, Kaye has provided services for Grammy award winning gospel artist CeCe Winans, Angie, Debbie, and Mom Winans, Congresswoman Eddie Bernice Johnson, Congresswoman Barbara Lee and a host of civic and business leaders. Kaye's honors and work lend proof to the scripture found in Proverbs 18:16, *"A man's gift makes room for him, and brings him before great men!"*

References

1. Browall, M, Gaston-Johansson, F, Danielson, E. (2006). Post-menopausal women with breast cancer. Retrieved from http://www.medscape.com/viewarticle/529158

2. The Economist. (2003, May 22). The beauty business, pots of promise. Special report. Retrieved from http://www.economist.com/node/1795852/print

3. Livingston, C., & Losee, S. (1997). *You've only got three seconds.* New York: Doubleday.

4. Retrieved from http://www.statisticbrain.com/hair-loss-statistics/

5. Centers for Disease Control. (2013). Head lice. Frequently asked questions. Retrieved from http://www.cdc.gov/parasites/lice/head/gen_info/faqs.html

6. American Hair Loss Association. (2013). Drug induced hair loss. Retrieved from http://www.americanhairloss.org/drug_induced_hair_loss/

7. BreastCancer.org. (2013, September 24). Cold caps. Retrieved from http://www.breastcancer.org/tips/hair_skin_nails/cold-caps

8. Waggoner, J., M.D. (2013). *Hormone harmony.* Dallas: My Sister's Keeper Press.

9. Khan, A. (2011, August 26). Surgeon General Regina Benjamin says a hairdo may deter exercise. Is she right? Retrieved from: *http://articles.latimes.com/2011/aug/26/news/la-heb-regina-benjamin-exercise-hair-style-20110826*

10. Waggoner, J., M.D. (2010) *Stress success.* Dallas: My Sister's Keeper Press.

11. Fleming-Dixon, J. (2012, November 6). The natural hair revolution will not be televised. Retrieved from http://forcoloredgurls.com/2012/11/the-natural-hair-revolution-will-not-be-televised/

12. Oprah.com. (2008, November 20). Beauty around the world. Retrieved from http://www.oprah.com/style/Beauty-Around-the-World/9

13. Office of Women's Health. (2013). Cosmetics and your health fact sheet. Retrieved from:
http://www.womenshealth.gov/publications/our-publications/fact-sheet/cosmetics-your-health.html

14. Smith, J. C. (1998). *Black heroes,* Detroit: Visible Ink Press.

15. Bundles, A. (2001). *On her own ground: The life and rimes of Madame C.J.Walker.* New York Washington Square Press.

General Reference:

Milady Standard Cosmetology. (2012). Clifton Park, New York: Cengage Learning.

Photo Credits

Blair Caldwell spazzphotography.com: Cover

Derrick Alonzo Brown: page - 16.

Hillary Bell: page - 17.

Tamara Crawford/ MaHogony Photography: pages - 130, 169.

Kendrick Goree/ Goree Enterprise goree-enterprises.com : pages - 146, 147.

Rod Warner Fitness: page - 104.

Hope Sierra Smith: page - 33.

C. Wilson Photography www.cwilsonphotography.com: all other photos.

"Beauty without character is worthless. I'll help you maintain your beauty; but the character development is up to you."

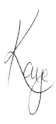